Supersize Your Single Mom Life

A Single Mom's Guide to Living Her Dreams

I0103330

Sunny Fungcap

chipmunkapublishing

the mental health publisher

Published by
Chipmunkapublishing
PO Box 6872
Brentwood
Essex CM13 1ZT
United Kingdom

http://www.chipmunkapublishing.com

Copyright © Sunshin Fungcap 2013

Edited by Laura Holliday

ISBN   978-1-84991-857-2

Chipmunkapublishing gratefully acknowledge the support of Arts Council England.

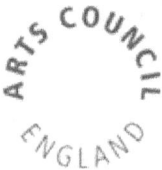

TABLE OF CONTENTS

Sunny Fungcap

Acknowledgments

Before anything, I would like to thank and acknowledge our divine creator for providing the inspiration to complete this book. Without the source of our being we would not be able to access information that proves so vital to our every day existence. I would also like to thank my daughter, Olivia, whom without having raised her, I would not have been able to say, *"Hey…I've been there."* She has been one of the greatest motivators in my life and along with any challenge, came a little bit of wisdom along with it.

I am grateful for the support of my family and found that every one of them provided a little something so that I may benefit and learn from my experiences as a mom. I would like to acknowledge those in my circle of personal relationships, who provided me with the strength, extra support, encouragement and inspiration I needed to move forward with my career.

Important groups in this whole process were the single mothers who contributed their opinions about their own experiences and also those outside this group who were so willing to admit to their own assumptions and perspectives on single motherhood. Thanks for being honest! Additionally, I would like to thank Patricia Benson in Polygon for her suggestions and feedback.

Lastly, I would like to recognize the benefit of any of the challenging experiences I have encountered in the past. These experiences made me stronger, more receptive, more proactive, and encouraged me to perceive things differently than I would have in the past.

Sunny Fungcap

Begin Your Journey by Evaluating Your Beliefs

Sunny Fungcap

Chapter 1
The "Single Mom" Taboo

At least once in her lifetime a single mother will hear the words: "You can't do it, you're a single mom" Or "Being a single mom, how would you find time or the money to do that?" Believe me, it is not the time a single mom lacks, it is the drive from within and the willingness to not accept what is often told by others who aren't where *they* want to be yet. It is a way for those individuals to put you in a sealed box you can never get out of. If you insist on remaining in that box you will be shielding yourself from a world of opportunities. If you don't take risks you won't know if you will ever be able to accomplish anything outside that box. You will be doing exactly what negative individuals expect your role should be: a single mom... and nothing else.

What is it about the phrase "single mom" that it is considered somewhat taboo? Why is single motherhood often automatically followed by the phrase "she deserves what she got" or "she needs a way out of her situation" and single fatherhood is followed by "he's doing a good thing" or "he is such a responsible person." Is one a form of punishment and the other a courageous sacrifice? Neither, of course! At least it doesn't have to be. Children are gifts that benefit from us, as well as we them. It is how the single mom or dad perceives their situation that determines their reality. Our perceptions usually come from what we accept from the media. Are we completely convinced that television is our most reliable source of reference to single parenthood? Don't live someone else's idea of you. Later, we will discuss more about the effectiveness of our own perceptions on outcomes.

Society however, has placed a stigma on single parents in general. The assumption is that in order for them to live their dreams, they must wait until children become old enough to fend for themselves. By this age, the parent is too tired and often ends up regretting that they didn't grab opportunities when presented to them at that time. This is especially the case for most single mothers who raise their children either alone on a full time basis or part time. Women may typically be seen as the primary caregiver, though more recently single fathers have taken on an increasing role.

Understand that not all these claims apply to single parents in every corner of the country, but it is common to believe that life as a single parent can make you feel a little delayed in getting where you want to go in life. The worst part is not that you aren't there, but that you have given up by accepting the generalization that single moms must sacrifice almost everything they desire or every dream to raise a child. Take it from me, if you sacrifice yourself, you won't be any good to that child of yours.

If you are open to hearing more about ways to achieve your goals as a single parent, then let's take a journey through myth-town shall we? Although many single parents move out of big cities since the cost of living is so high, New York City areas are swarming with independent single moms waiting or are already beating the odds. We can begin by tackling some of the myths that may keep the single mom stagnant.

Myth #1: "It's going to be too hard for you."
It isn't how hard. It's how far you are willing to go to reach it without compromising your child. (What is considered compromising to you?)

Myth #2: "You are putting your child second."

Just like the oxygen mask you must put on yourself first during a turbulent flight, take care of *you* so you can take care of your child. You *are* actually putting your child second if you don't take care of yourself emotionally, physically, financially, and spiritually.

Myth #3: "Don't let your child(ren) see you cry."

A child would be better off seeing how you pick yourself up from heartache and disappointment, as opposed to seeing an invincible super hero with the immortal power to resist feeling down about anything. Children need to learn recovery methods, not how to suppress tears. Though if you are the type to cry every time milk spills, consider the reaction you are teaching your child. Who do you think she will be modeling after when something quite minor occurs?

Myth #4: "Now that you have a weekend to yourself don't just sit home. Live a little and go out!"

Great! All you need is more mental activity and running around right? It isn't that going out with your friends isn't stress relieving, but let's face it, when was the last time you were able to be still and spend time doing the things you love alone? There is no reason to feel embarrassed if when you do get opportunities to be alone, you'd rather spend it solo. It is part of keeping a balanced life.

Myth #5: "Once your child grows to be a bit more independent, then do the things you've always loved doing!"

Don't let your child be the reason to not live your dreams, but rather, the motivation.

Myth #6: "Here's a guy for you. Hey at least he is single."

It doesn't seem to matter if he is rude, obnoxious and growing an extra toe does it? There are people out there who just want to play matchmaker for a single mom because well...he's a man right? Wrong. Single moms should not suddenly lower their standards because they think men will not date them if they are raising a child alone. Women also should not base their attraction for someone on what they themselves lack, but rather what they have to give. She will be stuck never feeling completely whole until he is around, and all the while her gut is saying he is not the man for her anyway. Who are we kidding?

Myth #7: "If your kid doesn't like him, dump him. You have to think of what your child wants first."

Someone once stated that a child usually senses if the person mom is dating is on the level or not. Their instincts are pretty much on point. I agree with this one hundred percent, however a child is not always acting out because their instincts are telling them the guy is trouble. It could be that the child thinks he or she may be losing your attention. A fear of "replacing dad" could be surfacing. It could be a number of things that may spark up tension between the three of you. Unless any type of abuse is suspected of course, the best thing for you to do would be to have a conversation with your child about what he or she is feeling and discuss a few options from there. Getting advice from former single moms about the way they handled dating before marriage may be a good idea.

The Two Step Ladder:

Now that we have addressed only a few of the many myths, what do you do now? You know in your heart that you can do more and would like to get there, but there are too many hurtles, such as finding and paying for babysitting, finding time to help your children with homework, and searching for valuable time with them. Many of the self-help books out there will tell you that it is a "process" and any great plan involves taking a series of steps. Well, guess what? Ninety percent of the time those authors are right. The ten percent comes from the idea that any sudden life change will result from something miraculously unexpected, also known as divine intervention, a miracle or some consider as "fate." The word *"process"* sounds long, but who says it has to be? A process can take as little as a week or as long as a lifetime. It is all up to you. You may not have to go through twenty-five steps to reach your goal. Ever heard of a two-step ladder?

The problem with steps is that nine times out of ten we don't know where to begin and which ladder to use. The one with the easy grip steps so you don't fall, the very tall, cylinder rung ladder that leaves you feeling accomplished, but drained by the time you get to the top *(which of course many people feel is the best route since they believe nothing worth it is without sacrifice)*, or the two step ladder, that although a little unsteady and you may need to do a little reaching at the end, is the quickest way to the goal. Then ask yourself these questions. Do you feel your child can yank the ladder right out from under you? Do you feel you will be putting too much attention on yourself that you missed their approach? Is it possible to get right back on after such a fall? We all go through this. The main difference a single mother may encounter, often times, is needing to make the decision alone. Don't be the one who passes right under the ladder. You will forget there was a goal up there in the first place.

Let's take a look at some steps you can take so that you begin to work on *you*. Topics about the self are often left towards the end of a book as if to say the first task an individual must do is to arrange their outside world and change the behavior of others. This is not the case here. Like the oxygen mask approach, work on you and your reality first. We will get to the illusion later.

If you have been living someone else's idea of who you should be then ask yourself, has that been working for you?

NOTES

CHAPTER 2
Life's Hectic

No matter what you want and how you believe you are going to get to where you want to be, life has a way of surprising you when you're not prepared. Once you have made a plan, life takes a turn. Don't take it as a cruel joke. Consider it a wakeup call to take control of your life and create your outcomes. If you know this already then the question is how do you know if what you are planning is where you truly want to be or has anything to do with your true life's purpose? The only way to know is to discover it. Try too hard and you miss it. Not quite getting it? Okay, here it is:

How many times in your life can you say you have actually heard a calling? If not much, in that case, you probably have too much mental activity going on to even hear what it is. According to the *Custodial Mothers and Fathers and Their Child Support consumer income report* from the U.S. census bureau August 2007, in the spring of 2006, there were about 13.6 million single parents of kids under twenty-one, and out of that amount how many do you think literally, on average, spends thinking about their child or something related to their child on a daily basis? My guess is almost all of them. Out of the mothers, about 44% have more than one child; so double the number of days. Even with changing fertility patterns today, the concerns are the same. These may sound familiar:

Thinking about...

> **Lunch money**
>
> **After school activities**
>
> **Teacher and other parent opinions**
>
> **Late child support deposit**
>
> **Step-parent issues**
>
> **Dinner for today**
>
> **Dinner for tomorrow**
>
> **Dinner for next month, and here's a good one: food to bring for the child's next classroom birthday party so you stay original!** *(Okay that may be a little over the top)*
>
> **Gas money to drive your child to various after school activities**

Here are some more that may sound familiar:

- Your child's peer pressure issues or concerns at school
- The events you know you want to and should attend because your child feels she is the only one without a parent there
- School plays
- Parent teacher conferences
- Field trip money letters sprung on you at the last minute
- Where to take them on the weekends
- How to fit time for your work that you take home
- When to finish that 2 week pile of laundry *(don't lie to yourself. If it's there just accept it)*
- When to actually shop for school clothes and supplies
- Thinking of how to discuss an important issue with your child
- Thinking of ways to avoid discussing an issue with your child
- When to schedule in doctor's appointments, immunizations, dental checkups
- Searching for day care
- Parent teacher conferences
- Wishing for at least one overnight care for...(*I'll leave that part up to you*)
- Thinking of where to run when your child's tantrum echoes from one end of the house to the other. There *is* nowhere to run. You just have to deal with it.... with love of course.

Those were just the minor concerns, demanding only a small amount of mental space. Here are the invaders:

- **When to move**
- **Where to move**
- **Should you move?**
- **Mortgage payments**
- **If you will even get child support at all**
- **Court fees**
- **How much distance to place between your child and the other custodial or non-custodial parent?**
- **How to encourage closeness between your child and the other parent**
- **Should you take that job?**
- **Should you quit your job and work at home?**
- **Should you start looking for another higher paying job?**
- **Should you get remarried now?**
- **Should you get remarried for security or love?**
- **If dating is even a possibility**
- **When should you talk about the next level with your mate?**
- **Should you involve your parents in your decision?**
- **Should you introduce a date to your child and if so when is the perfect time?**
- **Should you open up a college savings account now?**
- **Should you start a u-promise account?**
- **Is your 401k really for you or for your child's future?**

More, more, more! A single mom's mind is racing a mile per minute that there is no way possible to fit in a true rewarding life of her own, separate from or even including her child's needs, right? Wrong! Spare a bit more mental space for this question: *"Who do I choose to be and how can I get there without compromising my child(ren)?" or "What do I really desire to do and can I still involve my child?"*

Rarely, does someone stop to think initiating a plan to time-manage the above tasks begins with something as simple as this. There is so much a single mom must think about. The mental activity required is demanding, not only on her time, but also her energy. If single parents are so busy thinking how do they have time to do those things? It takes less exhaustion to do something while you love doing it than if you found little joy in it. Taking your child to a soccer game should be joyous right? Absolutely, but unfortunately it is more of something parents see as *having* to do rather than *wanting* to do. However, once you have begun doing the things you truly enjoy and take time out for yourself, you'll find that many tasks that used to be what you considered "your job," would be what you now call "your privilege." You then begin to see more tasks as "blessings" or "experiences" rather than routine tasks that make you believe you are on that familiar road to nowhere. You need to manage your life in your mind first before you can do it tangibly.

It is a challenge, however, to efficiently manage anything in your head without making room to imagine something you enjoy. Just like your body when you're at work, your mind also needs a break from the routine. Putting aside the whimsical cloudy and rosy-child-like images just for the sake of bringing out your inner-youth, imagining actually has a tangible purpose in your life. To attract what you desire!

The way you can begin doing this is by recognizing what attracts you. Keep this picture in your mind and *learn* to bring it to you! It's that simple! Picture the answers to those burning questions about your life in your mind, forcing the universe to respond the way you think. Be consistent with it.

Begin by taking out one sheet of paper and a pen. List your goals, numbering them from one to ten. Don't list them as questions. List them as answers or better yet, affirmations! For example:

- **I am a successful chef**
- **I own my own business**
- **I look, am, and feel physically fit**
- **I make more than (choose your amount but believe it)**
- **I am married to the man or woman I've always desired to have as a partner or I am happy as a single parent**
- **I have the self confidence I need to attain my goals and to be ambitious**
- **I have time to live my dream and raise my child the way I know best**
- **I travel to or around (_favorite place_) often or two times per year**
- **I am at my ideal weight**
- **I have a respectful and loving relationship with my child (ren)**

Affirmations can be said in various ways. You can simply state that you are thankful for the above or you can say that you are in the process of obtaining the goal. It just has to be believable to you.

Now, simply clear your mind by drawing in three

deep breaths that last seven seconds each before exhaling. These breaths will allow your mind to relax and clear, to gain focus and to draw in a divine life force that will bring on more inspiration the *more* you do it. Once you have taken the deep breaths, sit in a quiet place during the time you have alone and visualize the ten affirmations coming to pass. If too many other thoughts are getting in the way, simply take those three deep breaths again and start all over. Every set will become easier and clear out more residue from your mind. Do this for as long as you need to in order to picture them in your mind. Soft music without lyrics is always helpful if you choose to use it. Make this your routine and see it as laying the groundwork in order for you to physically get to where you are already seeing in your mind. Your universe will support and your body will do things that your mind calls it to do eventually and without you even realizing it at times.

Next, get one more sheet of paper out or, even better, find or purchase a dry erase board to hang up on the wall in your private room. Write the following phrases:

"What you think about the most will expand."
"If you complain, you will attract more of what you complain about."
"Feel the fear and do it anyway!"
"Don't hold in your tears or you will never get to the next emotion."

If you are looking at the last phrase as an emotion you just don't have time to feel, do not think you are doing yourself any favors and assume that you are being strong for your child. Think of crying as rain drops filling a bucket. There is only so much the bucket can take before it spills over. That bucket wouldn't have room for anything else until you drain it out. This is why so many women get through and over long-term relationships a lot quicker than most men do. Suppressing all tears in the beginning will leave you returning later once you have had enough of holding it in. Crying it all out in the beginning will provide you with the clarity you need to know what to do with yourself next. Don't hold it in! Also try to remember that you would not know what happiness meant without experiencing disappointments.

Now back to the three phrases.

It doesn't matter if you write the affirmations and the principles one hundred times or just once. It will be just as effective waking up one hundred mornings and looking at the one list each time. It will also be just as effective if you looked at it just once and simply reminded yourself daily. Putting it everywhere in your house will also have the same effect. It is not about the quantity, but your intention to have it work for you! The universe knows your intention.

Wherever you put the list, place it where you can read it each morning after you wake up. This approach will not only remind you of these principles and affirmations, but the words will also eventually resonate in your mind so that you become convinced that they are a part of your reality. You may find yourself reiterating the words to others with ambition and purpose and may react in a more positive manner. It will get you to not fixate on the negative that may be occurring in your life. Furthermore, learn the lessons you bring to yourself, or better yet, the meaning and purpose of a situation and then move on! Not learning it the first time will only re-attract the same or harder lesson sooner or later so you force yourself to learn it until you get it. This is a sneaky little trick in life people tend to miss coming, but it is something we all can avoid.

NOTES

If you feel lonely remember that God is a verb. It's difficult to feel love if you don't give it. If you offer it, you're saying you've owned it

NOTES

Chapter 3
Be Alone; Not Lonely

After feeling burned, following a long and life-altering relationship with an ex-mate, it is easy to fall into the thinking that there is nowhere to go but up. You are convinced that your next relationship will either be much better or you are bound to experience relationship-hell for life! The next relationship begins beautifully, only to find that it is going in the same direction, doesn't seem to be working and the burn is even worse than before. It is hard to believe, since the second relationship seemed perfect and a reward was expected for the horror you went through during the first relationship, but history seems to repeat itself doesn't it? Hence, the thinking that *"this always happens to me!"* or *"Why can't I find the right one?"* or *"I thought Karma would send me a reward for being the victim last time!"* If you think you're a victim, you are a victim always until that thought changes. The idea is to learn from the first one so the same experience and, more than likely, even worse isn't attracted back to you. It hits harder because the first time around you didn't learn so the lesson gets tougher. We are not being punished. We, as spiritual beings, only attract lessons so that we may discover the way out and make another choice. Though there is always an easier route, we tend to choose the way that gets us lost. Sometimes the choice is not about picking something entirely different, but picking a different way to see it.

Every relationship will involve two people playing the same roles, teacher and student. In other words, both have something to teach and both have something to learn. None of us are exempt no matter how good we think we are. If you come out of the first relationship assessing what it is you needed to get out of it, you will embrace what you had rather than regret it and, therefore, creating a door for the divine universe to bring you a fresh new and better experience with someone else or with the same person. Many times a single mom will find herself asking, "It has been a year already! Why haven't I found someone yet?" At the time of question, there is doubt and where there is doubt breeds negativity and there you have it. You have not embraced the learning experience long enough and quit three days before the new guy came. Now you have convinced yourself he isn't coming when he was just around the corner.

If there is more to learn in relationship class there will be more to go through, but it won't always end badly. How boring is it to end up with a partner whom you feel you have stopped learning from permanently? Where is the mystery? You might as well agree on everything! We pretend that we can only teach others, and refuse to learn from our partner so then we have the control. Relationships are not about control, but rather connecting with someone through the experience and discovering its purpose. We take the same approach with our children. We feel we have children only to teach them and think there is nothing that they can teach us.

Let's rewind a little. My intention is not to imply that each of us must go through life's relationships with a big question mark hanging over our heads. It is to emphasize that we learn as well as teach and that we can only do this by letting go of a struggling relationship so the true purpose of both partners can reveal itself. This applies whether the end result is marriage or permanent separation. Each lesson adds to who we are and creates character. Some of the more prominent figures in our lifetime have endured some painful learning experiences only to become great teachers. The difference is that at some point in their lives they had made the decision to consider their series of "painful" experiences as speed bumps they've successfully driven over rather than ladders too high to climb.

Since the role of a single mom is a tough one, every new idea seems like a new task, a new job, and just another thing to think about. The idea is to not think so hard or you will eventually think yourself into doubt! Let go of that prison and give yourself enough internal pampering to get the ball rolling for you. Before you know it your world of relationships will reflect exactly what you've always desired.

NOTES

*"Knowledge is learning something new every day.
Wisdom is letting go of something every day."* --Zen
Proverb

NOTES

Chapter 4
Travel Like You Have The Time

Here is a riddle for you. During times of stress, what is the first thought in every single mom's mind, yet the last thing thought to actually do? That's right! See? You thought of it…Vacation! We want vacation from work and humdrum routine, from physical strain, and emotional drainage. Often travel isn't taken as seriously as it is taken in our minds. We can say to ourselves a billion times that we will be going to Tahiti next year, but what part of your body will make the first move towards that trip, your hands to purchase the ticket online or your feet to urge you towards your boss to request your vacation? A great number of single moms tend to put off travel plans for reasons such as not having enough money, being tied to a work schedule, lack of babysitting, or not being able to find someone to fly with. This half of her is thinking of every excuse in the book to keep her from actually going. The other half is patiently waiting. A lot of times these thoughts come to mind first when contemplating taking time to go away: *I'll have time to go away someday. I have a child to raise first. What would I do with him while he is this young? It's not practical and I wouldn't be a responsible parent.*

Traveling to an area much different than what you are used to often inspires creative thinking and original ideas. Creative and new is how you will want to experience life after the boring routines you encounter day in and day out. If travel is on your mind and on your affirmation list, whether it is for a specific job or simply for leisure then begin your journey with the following simple task. Find all the magazines you can around your home. You can purchase a few from the store, print pictures from the Internet or search through newspapers. Magazines tend to work the best because of the quality of the photographs. Cut out the pictures of places where you would like to go or look for ones that are similar in landmarks and features. You can do the same for other goal-related pictures. As juvenile as it may appear, try placing these pictures either on your wall or against your mirror, where it can be viewed daily.

Sometimes going back to how we used to create during our childhood is the best place to start. Believe that this approach will allow for the pictures to creep its way into your mind, finding a permanent nesting place to reside in. How quickly it creeps is up to you and your persistence to never let the dream go! Wherever you find a peaceful haven, find the picture and post it on several places inside whatever room you are in the most. Sometimes it isn't the bedroom for single moms. It might be the living room where there is a sofa, the first sight of a resting place once arriving home from an unbearable day. The pictures will also help you to visualize the places you want to go to. Again, your thoughts will form its way into reality in some shape or form. This can work for other purposes, such as building your dream kitchen, buying the perfect boat, or landing a great job.

I recall a conversation with a relative of mine who spoke about the irony of his last relationship with beautiful women. He claimed that for two years he woke up to a posted magazine picture of this woman, whose features he had admired and found unique. He said that he did not put the picture up for any other reason than to admire her beauty. An article under her picture read of a short summary of likes and dislikes for the purpose of advertising men's cologne. One evening he arrived at a hotel to hear a speaker at a convention pertaining to his business, only to have met a women looking almost exactly like the model in the magazine photo. Of course, she wasn't her clone, but after brief introductions and a conversation, he had realized that this woman was very similar in her likes and dislikes. It was an eerie experience for him, yet somewhat magical. They dated for years following their encounter. Looking back, it dawned on him that he might have thought he was simply posting a magazine photo of a beautiful woman, when actually he was keeping it there with the intention of attracting her in his life. Sometimes you have no idea what you've wanted all along. The same method applies to the ideal vacation spot, whether it is an escape to Hawaii, to upstate New York, or to a good friend's beautifully- landscaped patio deck for the weekend.

There will always be that person who says, *"Right now you have priorities."* Of course you do. We all do and one of them is to take care of you. Many times we tend to believe that priorities lie in the external because when things outside of us go right then we *appear* to be doing well or we conclude we are doing well only based on standards set by others. What should actually take precedence is the need to feed your soul with what you've been urging for so you can be the person you need to be to work diligently on those external priorities.

It is okay to feel that your child comes first in everything you do, however there is a difference between *thinking* of her first and *putting* her first. For example, let's say you are arguing with your nine-year-old child because she has been acting out at school. You are constantly snapping back at her and the two of you are bickering about her constant request to attend her most anticipated event ever that you do not have time, or the money for.

You have two choices, you can *put* her first by giving in to her request and simply finding the means to make it happen because you just don't feel like dealing with it right now or you can *think* (which is really putting her first in a proactive way) of her first by finding a way to help her learn the art of compromising during a time when you just don't have the means. A possible solution would be for your nine year old to go next time or to go this time, but only to stay part of the time. The fact that you did not give in to her full request shows that you care about what she is learning from this. If she knew she deserved disciplining and you never did it, eventually she will conclude that you just don't care. You are not trying to be her friend more than you are trying to be her mom.

Putting your child first means you must take care of you so that you can take care of her or him. Doing something you truly enjoy *is* a priority. Avoid thinking of leisure time as selfish or extravagant. Also avoid thinking that someone else is just fortunate for the opportunity to travel. There are always opportunities, but they can be blocked with the belief that a person has to be fortunate in some way. You are fortunate in many ways. The only thing that sets you apart is your determination to seek the right channels and the negative thinking that blocks them from appearing in your life. It is this sort of thinking that gets you to automatically think of vacation and traveling as something you will do "one day" while everyone else is scheduling days on a routine basis. There is nothing written anywhere that dictates that single moms never snorkel, roller blade, ski, join world dance competitions, model, perform on stage, or do karate on the side or full time. In fact, one of my old friends was a state champion in Karate, opened up a school and is going to law school part time. No, she did not come from money. How did she do it? She didn't know she couldn't! After she made up her mind, she did not surround herself with people who she knew would constantly remind her that she didn't have time, she didn't have the skills, she couldn't do it, and that she was being selfish. Now, her child is learning this as well. Teach your child to strive and believe. It is our belief system that allows us to continue moving forward, knowing goals can be achieved under any circumstance.

NOTES

Chapter 5
Get to Your State of Being

One point that must be made is that what you focus on does expand. Many people believe blocking or avoiding thoughts about what they desire will help them not to focus on what they are lacking in their lives. This is denying the part of you that actually makes life work. No one is saying to think about what you're missing, but rather to picture what you know you can have if you used your will to obtain it. Picturing your goals alone doesn't give you what you desire, that is why we have a physical body to use as a vehicle to get to where you want to be, not go...BE! (When you *Do* certain things, you will learn to *perform* the small and incremental deeds that will get you to the attitude, *Being happy etc,* so that you can attract what you desire and so that you are pleased). Though visualizing your goals while attempting to reach those happy feelings aroused by the scenes in your mind does guarantee you an open door, so that you may walk in and grab it! You cannot do this however if you do not use some of the valuable time that you do have to yourself and use it accordingly. You will get to your goals, but pushing the methods to get there aside will leave you feeling delayed, unless of course you win the lottery! Even after winning the lotto, however, an inner-nagging sensation may still linger within you. The universe can only respond to the way you feel and think about yourself and your ability to attain your goals. You aren't the passenger. You are actually the driver who can control and steer your feelings to help you reach your goal, but it depends on your thoughts about getting to your destination.

Remember to perform these tasks, either on an on-going basis, or at least until you have opened a window of discovery and realized where you really want to go and what you desire to be. Continue to allow your desires to manifest before your eyes. In a nutshell, fulfilling your dreams is about being at a positive state first before you can really do anything to reach them. While you are trying to resolve something with all your might, you will continue to perform with your inside-self nudging you to take a different course or telling you this is not where you really want to be. This is what our society calls "something missing." That something missing is not anything or anyone outside yourself. When your partner goes on a business trip and you continue to feel something "missing," it means that you depended on that person to provide you with that feeling, that happy state you want to reach. When you work at a relationship without working on yourself first, you are only trying to fix something outside yourself when the results depend on how you are being inside. What perspective are you taking on a certain situation? Are you sure you are not overreacting with anger and blame? See if there is a way to resolve those feelings and see if the situation changes. Be whole and attract! Don't fear and chase! Do you recall the phrase, *"Follow your dreams?"* Don't chase them. Chasing them only says to the universe that your dreams are *always* just out of reach and therefore, adds the resistance preventing dreams from being fulfilled This doesn't mean be lazy. Following them means by becoming a whole person, finding your true divinity within yourself, you will attract the opportunities that will present themselves to you and you will know where the doors are that lead you to your greatest desire!

Opportunities are always presented to you. Fear hates to choose and it never seems to win. So why choose fear?

NOTES

Chapter 6
Entrepreneurship for the Single Parent

Owning your own business is quite an accomplishment for a single parent. The time and money it takes to start up a business is normally beyond what the single parent has in his or her possession, unless money is inherited. If your family has left savings in your name then only part of this book applies to you. In any case, congratulations! If you haven't already, you would like to be your own boss and raise your child simultaneously. Are people telling you your nuts yet? There are many single parent entrepreneurs who found ways to manage their time with their children. In fact, many found ways of allowing the business to give them more quality time with their kids.

Remember, regardless of the time it takes to run a business, you ultimately call the shots. Of course eventually you will expand and delegate, take on a few employees or independent contractors. You may also decide that the best decision-maker is someone other than you, but for the initial stages you open a business you are passionate about, just make sure it continues to be just that...what your passionate about, otherwise it really becomes just work. When a business mission and vision turns into something other than what it was initially intended to be, you have literally relinquished your rights to the business itself or possibly to a partner who has a different vision and mission in mind. It is as if you are working for someone else. Rather than you scheduling based on your desire of how you want your business to operate, you are scheduling to meet deadlines you've never anticipated and to distinguish more fires than you can handle. This will never give you the time you desire with your family. In fact, the time you do manage to get, will not be chosen by you, but by your customers, clients, consumers etc...

It is essential to always go back to the original reason why you started the business or organization. Just like life, you are always going back to its purpose. When you do this you put things into perspective when having to make tough decisions. Especially for professionals who opened a business with the intent of performing something of service to the community, it is easy to get lost and to forget why the business was established in the first place as it starts to grow. It is just as easy to become so overly "service-oriented" that you are not generating enough income to barely break even. You start to offer so much leeway because you feel guilty asking for people to pay on time when you are the person supposedly trying to make a difference in someone's life. Money does not always have to remain at a distance from a passionate entrepreneur simply wanting to offer something to the world. If anything, often single parents who own businesses know they have to be very passionate about what they do, since they acknowledge the time and financial investment it will consume. Therefore, it is their passion that drives them to decide to invest the money they were going to stash away for little Taylor's first year of college, towards the growth of the business. The decision weighs heavily because you have to make a choice between providing partial security for your child's future educational needs, and financial success you will push to get through your business. Which one can you control? What risk are you willing to take? Whether in business or life, without risk, you miss certain opportunities. So ask yourself if it is serving you and your child to play it "safe."

Before venturing off into the unknown, make sure you do your research on the business you are planning to start. Understand the differences between having a corporation and operating as a sole-proprietor. It is common for single parents to start as sole-proprietors since operating costs, managing, maintaining overhead and equipment and other supplies, all come from and performed by them in the beginning. Understand the tax benefits and know how you can separate your business and personal life. Even if you love your career, do not neglect the time you need for yourself. Question if the time you enjoy most is the time spent growing your business. If it isn't, you are not doing it any favors, nor yourself and your child if you are in the office all weekend and throughout the week, since we can see that overachieving in one area *(the business)* can leave you deficient in other *(social and family life)*.

If you are serving others in some way after you have obtained some training it is best to choose a niche that you can display, discuss, and practice. The reason for this is that, unless you are starting with business partners or receiving help of some kind, marketing too many services at once tends to leave you feeling scattered and unfocused. You find yourself overwhelmed by your career, the feeling creeps back into your home life, and your child ends up being your sounding- board. You diminish your quality and effective time towards yourself, your child, and your business because you are so busy pausing to collect yourself and probably most of your paperwork. If you have the passion to offer many services through your business, then strategize one or two at a time and use your resources from the people you meet at functions and networking events. There are a lot of free networking events and groups to join online to enhance your business.   Remain proactive, but you will need some rest to recharge and re-gain some inspiration.

Starting a Non-Profit Business

Having the idea to start a nonprofit is rewarding in itself since the incentive usually comes from your inner self, inspiring you to serve and connect with others. There is a sense of fulfillment on earth when you are living a life helping others, but if it becomes overwhelming you will only drive your nonprofit to the ground and you will not serve the way you intended. Starting a nonprofit requires a team of people whom you feel can contribute to your cause in some way. Many single parents have friends they can socialize with, but because they are often so caught up in surviving at most that once they are motivated to start a project for a cause they can hardly find the network of people and resources to aid them in their quest. They have spent most of their time serving their children and may have put off furthering their education, that there was barely enough and time or means to build any type of network to help with a dream.

It is imperative that at any time in your life, whether you are raising a two-year old or a sixteen-year old, if you decide that you want to start a business or nonprofit that you practice the art of allowing, meditation, and ask our divine source for guidance on how to begin. If you delay these important tasks, you may not have a clear goal and direction in mind and you may be making business decisions that are counterproductive to your intentions. If you are confident in your direction then you are able to lead and guide others, and align your actions with you vision and mission.

You will find yourself going to the library and noticing the exact titles for the questions you have about starting a nonprofit. You may meet the right people on the street, or someone may offer an idea or be of some assistance to your cause. It is worth it to take the time to do what is necessary for your inner being before you can serve your clients, not to mention an entire community.

Protecting Yourself From Lawsuits

I am not an attorney so I cannot advise you on the legal aspects or ramifications of certain business decisions, however I can suggest that you always seek ways to protect yourself as an entrepreneur. Since money may at times be an issue in your personal life, you will want to separate your business dealings from your personal to a large degree. My suggestion would be to find qualified legal assistance to aid you in the process of protecting your own name from lawsuits against your business name. This is why it is imperative to work with a solid team. Just because you have survived serving a child alone for many years doesn't mean you have to serve your business alone as well.

Inspiration From Your Child

Ultimately, you will discontinue your attempts to grow the business if what originally inspired you starts to dwindle. Since you are more likely than single people without children, starting or doing this by yourself, you are constantly having to recall and go back to what inspired you in the first place. This is exactly what you should be doing since most among the best companies and organizations begin with inspiration, while others that fail start for any reason but. I recall several moments when something new has begun in my life, that it was not furthered or initiated without the inspiration from my daughter. It may have been something she said or did, but somehow she came through without even knowing it. Since she inspired me, she became my incentive and not the "in spite of" in my career life. I used this phrase less: *"I am starting this, in spite of having a child to take care of,"* and more of *"She has inspired me even more."*

Chapter 7
Laws to Live By

Spiritual development is integral to our daily functioning as human beings living in this planet. Due to our individual "challenges" we face on a routine basis, we constantly have to remind ourselves to seek ways to remember who we truly are, to recall happiness and how to get back to having peace of mind. Essential laws exist to remind us that happiness is indeed a choice, but there are also reasons why events occur and reoccur in our lives. Part of our spiritual development involves the emphasis of using practical exercises to help us become more enlightened individuals. It is a way to access the tools we already posses inside of us so that we may reap the benefits of rewards we were entitled to all along. Single parents especially, may feel disconnected from the rest of the world, as if to imply that a person raising a child solo is so uncommon.

There are so many ways to reconnect with the universe, but this doesn't mean we were ever apart from it. We do things to block this connection and forget how to access what it takes to obtain what we truly desire out of life. *Linda Capobianc, PhD*, an instructor and Holistic Health Practitioner at the *Holistic Healers Academy in NJ*, provided insightful thoughts regarding essential laws to remember, including a very important way of achieving desired results in life: applying the **Laws of the Universe.** In our search for enlightenment, there are laws that, if applied, force us to change our perspectives and way of life to bring about more successes. Very often we strive to seek help to fix one area in life, but neglect the other. Some people think that when they feel they are missing something in their life they can compensate by overachieving in another area and, thereby, allowing the stronger part to represent who they are. The **Law of Balance** teaches us that a healthy life is a balance between all the areas that make us who we are. If we are overachieving at work, our social life may suffer. We may have really exciting social lives, but may be depleting ourselves of quiet time. Very practical energy healing exercises exist to help us recognize what balance feels like.

The Law of Choice helps us to remember that we are responsible for the outcomes in our lives. Do we choose to look at situations differently or are we victims of every encounter? Simply changing a perspective has the power to alter a situation, but it is the choice of the individual to change what they do not feel good about in life. However, we cannot throw caution to the wind just yet. We must choose our thoughts and words wisely because we just might get what we *decided* on. Notice I said, "decided" and not "wish," while wishing alone does not attract what we want, but deciding means what is desired has been chosen and if it has been chosen, it already exists. This **Law of Attraction** is an important means to success. It helps us to remember that we are the drivers and not just the passengers. We control the outcomes to the events in our lives. Often times a single mom will utter the words, "I can't, and that's just reality." No, that is *your* reality, and you would be surprised to see how perceiving a situation differently can change an outcome. For example, what is the first thing you think of when some says to you, "You're a single mom." Did you think, *I'm at a disadvantage somehow...I think.* At least that is what the person's words implied right? If you think you are at a disadvantage than you probably feel sad or frustrated.

You are at a disadvantage if you are feeling thinking and therefore feeling that way. No one is there to argue with you since you have made up your mind and declared it to yourself.

Furthermore, when we choose, we should remember that not seeing results right away doesn't mean to quit minutes before the miracle, which, by the way is relative to what many people often think of as the arduous, **Law of Process.**

How we perceive the process to get to the goal is just as important as the goal itself. We may decide the process we are going through is something bad, have doubts, and then it changes. We think we know where we are headed in the process instead of simply being in the present moment; therefore interfering with what would have been desired results. We must let go of deeply held energies from the past that may interfere with our perception of a new process and don't get too attached to specific expectations. Trust and expect that all things will work out overall and in divine order.

Think of the **Law of Cause and Effect**, since for every effect there is a cause. Our doubts caused the effects of changed outcomes. To elaborate on this concept, we use the example of treating an illness. Very often we treat our symptoms of an underlying condition. We are prescribed medication that have side effects, and therefore treat this. We do not treat the cause, but the effect. Thought follows this as well. When we are experiencing a situation that does not agree with us, we should recall the initial thoughts we had about the issue. The thoughts precipitated the effect, but we can always change them by controlling our thought pattern throughout the day.

A very significant way to do this is to see love in the entire universe, by applying the **Law of**

Compassion. Seeing love breeds a thought process that allows love to return in abundance. Changing a perspective on what another person is sending you may allow the situation to turn around.

The loneliness a single mom can feel at times will drive her to think she must protect herself from love so she doesn't get hurt, but all the while this protection is keeping love from returning in a healthy fashion; the way she truly wants it. Many times, the single mom will protect herself from true love from a wonderful man, but will all too easily accept much less because she feels it is what she deserves or it is all she feels she can get considering her circumstances of being a single parent. We are all connected to each other, so love is bound to return. This also means applying forgiveness as often as possible. Not letting go will hurt you just as much, if not even more than the other person. We are co-creators in our universe and can change a situation around, but we have to believe that we are not born to be sad.

The **Law of Happiness** entitles us to a birthright to be happy. We are constantly seeking happiness maybe because we know down deep it is natural feeling that belongs to us. Creating a list of cues to help remember what it is like to be happy will bring out the same feelings.

Just as the **Law of Action** represents, take action to recreate the life you want. It is to our advantage to have handy a list of cues to help remember what it feels like to be happy. For instance, say another driver cuts you off on the road during your morning commute to work. Following this your coffee spills and creates a puddle on the passenger seat. At the same time you remember you have a special evening meeting tonight that will have you miss a talent show you promised your child you would attend. You are already late to work and your aggravation continues to escalate. STOP! "Beach, Sunshine, last night's date!" Whatever works, think it and say it out loud if you have to. Maybe these are not the words that work for you however, it is a good idea to be honest with yourself and choose what really gets you excited. If your favorite cheese dish does it for you, so be it. I wouldn't advise stopping cold on the road. Just slow down on to the shoulder and breathe to reduce your tension and start all over using the cues. If you are already late a couple of minutes more will not make a difference, but it will affect your state of mind, which will eventually have an impact on the events of the day. This is guaranteed. Wouldn't you rather be late and see that your boss's negative feedback did not affect your state of mind as oppose to being late and having your work reflect the frustrations you feel?

If you go to a well known book store, you may find countless books entailing the art of applying the law of attraction, attraction principles, get what you want in five days or less, breath your way to success, don't want it and it will want you! Well it is simple really. There is not as much work to it as there is choice. In fact there shouldn't be work to it all. Although, all the books on this topic contain information vital to maintaining a fairly pleasant existence here on earth, it really comes down to what you already own, but could change, which is thought, desire, hope and belief. If you desire to lose a significant amount of weight, you have to begin by ascertaining in your mind that you are in the process of shedding pounds (or calories, or inches). Better yet, thank the Universe for the weight loss, as if to say you are choosing that outcome rather than choosing to be overweight. At that point the universe has no choice, but to comply. The events in your life will support you losing the weight.

Think of the universe as a giant bowl of Jell-O and you are in the center dug deep in that Jell-O. The Jell-O is so soft you are able to mold it in any shape or form you choose and let's all hope we choose what we desire, otherwise you will not have the experience you enjoy. If you were outside that Jell-O looking at it, molding it from above the bowl you could still shape the Jell-O, but from the perspective so far off and away, creating distortion and misperception of what is actually going on inside. Not too many examples can clearly convey the wonderment of how life can truly be, given that we attempt to become more aware of how much control we have over our circumstances.

Often times I find single mothers, more than married moms, worrying about weight loss after they have had one or two children. Whether married or not being a parent has its own challenges, but the ones single parents face alone on top of having to create the agenda just suitable for an effective weight loss routine can be a bit too much to bear. This has been the argument and the excuse. Weight loss and overall health maintenance has been secondary to the world of issues surrounding parenthood. It is not too often, however, that a single mom will convey that she has chosen to start focusing more on taking care of herself. This can easily happen to a single parent.

Have you ever experienced moments when you have had to make so many decisions you could no longer focus? You literally felt as if your mind was about to explode. Have you ever had one of those days when you were actually presented with so many great options that what many would think is an advantage, is actually too many choices to think of? The reason this happens is that regardless of the conditions you are surrounded with, whether it *forces* you to make a decision or *allows* you to choose between numerous desirable options, if there are too many, you find it difficult to move forward because your mind is experiencing too many thoughts at once. It is as if you were walking into a room surrounded by all your preferred flowers, they are all very exquisite, but which one do you choose if you can only pick one? So now you are absorbing each flower, using four or five your senses simultaneously. If someone reminded you that all you had to do is know before you walk in that all of your favorite flowers were in that room already and you could walk in and choose one, it would be easier wouldn't it? You would have already chosen one in your mind and then very confidently walk straight to it and grab it. Remain confident that the flower you chose was the best one for you at that time. Being clear-minded is the same as having a knowingness of a choice and then experiencing what you choose without distraction. You are now okay with the fact that there are so many flowers to choose from because you already made that choice before you walked in. Everything is already there for you to make that choice and be grateful for it ahead of time.

It is ironic that a number of women frequently find it counterproductive for a man to claim to only be capable of handling one thought at a time, when in fact it is what we should be striving to do.

This is how the law of attraction works. You simply make a choice, know it is out there to take it and proactively follow the opportunities that lead you to it. I did say follow, not chase. Chasing too hard presents the idea that you don't have it and fear you never will. This idea applies to people *and* objects. Isn't it better to say, "pursuing a bachelor's degree" on your resume rather than "chasing a bachelor's degree?" The degree is already there, so why would you chase it?

With divine support, simply move towards it as if it has been right there waiting for you. The path mentioned above, in this case, represents all the events the universe gives you; all of those funny little *synchronicities* we sometimes call "coincidences" supporting what you chose so that you can get to that outcome. In the case of weight loss, you choose your ideal weight in your mind, know that your desired result is available to you and obtainable (believe it), and by holding on to those thoughts, you see how life will support a path to shedding those pounds. You may see it through attracting opportunities to meet people who just happen to give you the best weight loss advice, joining a program that you suddenly can afford, or suddenly feeling inspired to exercise more. You see you will reduce the "struggle" and "trying" to make things work, however, it is implied that the struggle is required because we do not make it easy for ourselves. We shut our own doors. Especially in the single parent world, where there are so many excuses to choose from: *"I don't have the time, I have Billy" "I don't have a partner to jog with..." "I don't have a partner because no one can deal with the fact that I have a kid. It has nothing to do with the way I take care of myself..." "I don't need to eat anything for dinner tonight, as long as my kid eats, my conscious is served."* (yeah, but not your body). *"I can't afford an exercise mat, a Pilates program, healthy food, and I definitely can't afford to waste time on a walking regime...I'm too busy." "I feel guilty, like I am spoiling myself by spending a little extra on the adult health snacks this week when I should be thinking of how to spend this extra cash for my kid."*

We fool ourselves into believing that there is always a door ready to close as soon as an opportunity arises, and then of course...it does! We just said it would, *didn't we*? We could stand in front of a mirror affirming one hundred times that we are twenty pounds less than we actually are, and if we believe the opposite of that affirmation while saying it, the desired result will never come to fruition. If a mother truly believes she doesn't have time because of Junior, but affirms all day that she does simply because she heard that one must "speak it into existence" the opposite will happen just because her actions will demonstrate what she believes, not what she says. Her anxiety about not having the time and attempting to resolve it based on fear will simply produce results that come from just that, her fears. This is the "work" we put ourselves through. It's not necessary, but we do it and this is what we call into our lives and define as learning experiences. It starts from the desire to change where you want to go, what you want to be and what dreams you desire to experience. Believe it and your life will demonstrate that there are not as many obstacles to single motherhood as there are opportunities! For more practical guidance on this concept, you can read the attraction list at the end of this chapter.

"Murphy's Law"

"Anything that will go wrong will." Is that the saying? "Murphy's Law" is not a natural law. It is only in terms of how *we* commonly see events happening in our lives. The universe does not exist to punish us and the angels are not sitting back in heaven laughing and pointing at us, saying, "You think your human is bad? Get a load of mine..." No one is playing a joke on us, no one aside from ourselves anyway.

It does seem like that sometimes though doesn't it? Especially, according to many single parents out there, since most would have never thought they would end up being a parent on the solo track. In fact there are clubs and organizations that exist solely on the premise of resolving the "Murphy's Law" conundrum. The solution is simply this: to recognize the laws of the universe and remember the law of attraction. Be aware of what you say and what you attract. In other words, be careful what you wish for. Your words are very powerful, but more so your thoughts. I remember once when I was years younger, before I grew into my career, I had bought a lottery ticket and, while holding it firmly, prayed to God that the amount of the ticket would double. It sure did! I won a whole two bucks! The ticket price was a dollar and I asked for the amount to double, so guess what? It did. Then I realized I never asked for the winning amount to double. Although that is not the best metaphor and I wouldn't suggest buying one hundred lottery tickets to debunk this theory, it is simply a small illustration of what could happen if you are not truthful and specific about what you desire to have.

If you do what truly identifies you then you are on the right track. This is why more and more people today are working on "centering" themselves to align what they think, feel and do so there is no conflict and confusion about the outcome they have attracted from the universe. "Mind, body and spirit" is not a just phrase used in some new age program. It is a three part being that in every moment seeks to become one so that all outcomes are exactly what we actually call forth. We tend to lie to ourselves and deny what is in the heart or ignore the mind and focus on the body. Either way, we confuse ourselves and wonder why results are not what we anticipated when we worked so hard. It is that simple. "Murphy's Law" is our perception and what we ultimately conclude when we aren't aware of this. It is essential not to have

Example: Find **what is sexy about you** and **use it** *naturally*. Batting your eyelashes may not work, but if you know you have pretty eyes, look at that person across from you, while you are discussing "go green!"

13. **Don't** feel the need to **talk *all* the time**. Sometimes it appears it is more about the need for **attention** than speaking with true purpose.

14. **Have goals** and focus on them. When you have no goals in life, when someone you love goes away for a while, you feel like **something is missing**. That something isn't them. That something **is what's in you.**

15. **Don't overachieve** in one area leaving the **other one neglected**. Seek balance.

16. Develop an **active routine** either through exercise, sport, or an activity for leisure not accompanied by toxic consumptions. Example: Belly Dancing, yoga, walking, or simply going out the house more often.

NOTES

Be the change you want to see happening in your life

NOTES

Chapter 8
A Healthy You is a Healthy Yours

Your child's life, your social life, your parenting skills, your mental state and career are only some of the many aspects affected by what you eat. As an advocate for natural healing, I have encountered many people inquiring about additional supplements to take to heal ailments caused by a great number of toxins. As a life coach, I am faced with inquiries about ways to improve a person's lifestyle, love life and career. Often times I recognize right away following a questionnaire about a person's general lifestyle habits that a change in types of food may be one way to go. Sessions with clients may entail discussing ways to maintain using practical healing techniques, which is often only half successful if the individual insists on eating foods so toxic to the body. Well what do you know! It really does boil down to those cheeseburgers eaten everyday during your lunch hour. Go figure. As a team builder, I seem to have the most challenge with audience members who cannot last through a sitting activity because they are so tired from the meal they just consumed. We have all gone through it; what many may refer to as, you know…the "*itis*?"

A meal consisting of fruits and vegetables may be of the same quantity and density as an intense red meat meal containing large percentages of unhealthy carbs, protein, and fat and, *whatever it is on your plate you cannot describe.* Though, the former will most definitely leave you feeling more satisfied than the latter. Knowing the best combination of food to eat throughout the day and a good caloric ratio will profoundly affect your mental state, digestion and overall physical capacity, and decision-making skills, thereby resulting in more feelings of fulfillment and ease when you return home.

Let's take a common scenario in a single mom's life and link it to the above concept. At some point in a single mom's life she will feel that the ideal version of a day off from work is a day spent lounging around in the house. As mentioned earlier in the book, it is recommended that "you" time is taken and cherished, even if it is to stay home and do nothing. Although, imagine what the "you" time would be like if you had the energy that allowed you to take advantage of your indoor and outdoor environment to a greater extent. Either way, "you" time is not spent reflecting on what could have or should have been, but rather how the day can be enjoyed. Lethargy can have a saddening effect on the mind and ultimately, the heart. Having no energy can make a beautiful day seem like a rainy one. A rainy day, in human perception, is like a cue reminding you of an unhappy memory. Unhappy thoughts lead to unhappy feelings if you think about it enough.

You have a choice to combine your foods to work with your body; to allow it to consume what it was designed to consume. If the choice is too hard to make and you often find yourself *almost* there than *actually* there, then there are ways to help you reach that point.

Many individuals have sought out hypnotists to lose weight, thereby allowing the power of suggestion to change unwanted behavior such as overeating or digesting the wrong combination of foods. People seek out doctors for prescribed aids, nutritionists for counseling and menu planning, and holistic consultants for advice about natural products to help them lose weight. You can find success to some degree by seeking out any of the above, however nothing will help if you do not place health in your list of daily priorities. The nutritionist, the counselor, the coach, the doctor, nor the hypnotist can help you if you do not want it. It is first up to you to decide.

Health does not only deteriorate because of poor food choices and lack of exercise, but also due to lack of activity in what you are passionate about. Though you have to remember that if you recognize this lack and try to work on what you are passionate about (i.e. career), you could still be left feeling as if something is missing because it doesn't work to over achieve in one area, leaving another area of your life neglected and under-achieved. If you succeed in your career, you may look back and realize you have neglected your health, your love life or, your worst-case scenario, your child's well being.

The healthiest person is a very balanced person and vice versa. The ultimate achievement is balance and that is where you feel most at peace. A practical approach to achieving balance is to become aware of all the areas in your life you desire fulfillment and work on all of them, moderately. Working on one too much, will leave you working on the other too little and you will feel as if you are missing something eventually. Going for mother of the year will probably win you the model PTA mom award, but then you have gotten very little sleep because of all you managed to do for your child, the students, the parents and the PT Association. Then you wake up the next morning dreading to go to the job you despise and come home wishing you can show your award to another living adult, but you were too busy to speak to any of your friends over the past year. You got your achievement and it is something to be proud of, but there is no balance. Therefore, as rewarding as it is to be mother of the year, the feeling diminishes when you realize there is something you have neglected.

Any part of you that you neglect leaves you feeling sad because your soul thrives on completeness and wants you to experience what it experiences. Remember, these are the nudges you feel when you say to yourself, "I feel like something is missing" or "I feel like there is more to life." When someone says they feel at peace somehow, normally it is because they have achieved some level of balance in their lives by working on all areas to some degree and by striving for completeness. The little balance is enough however, to feel joy for a long time. Exercise and good food choices are ideal, but once you have reached a plateau, which we all have in our routines when it seems as if the plan just stop working, it is best to try something new. Aside from only starting a different diet or modifying your workout routine, perhaps breathing techniques, tai chi, meditation, fasting, or yoga?

Yoga

Yoga is widely used and has numerous health benefits. This is especially so for the single mother, although the practice of yoga is advantageous to anyone capable of performing the exercises. Yoga can prevent pain, strengthen muscles, improve balance, improve breathing, reduce stress, improve sex life, increase relaxation, improve confidence and posture, and help an individual to become more aware of what his or her own body can do. Ironically, some people are not aware they are performing Yoga also to circulate and free energy. Since energy is in and all around us, we are obligated to know more about how to make it function purposefully and to our advantage, especially when it comes to developing a health schedule.

Various Yoga styles, such as Hatha and Kundalini, exist for different people, therefore individuals of all ages and sizes do it. It is also something that can be done with your child at home or in a yoga instruction class. It can be entertaining, spiritually uplifting, and educational to children as well. Often times, children are not aware of how flexible they are until they have tried it.

The following figures are a combination of yoga/chi-kung poses for energy and stress relief. Know that there is a reason why yoga, tai chi, Qigong and other centering exercises demand tranquil surroundings, and you would be surprised to know that individuals on a fixed routine seeking enlightenment will tune out any distraction, while using all that their environment offers to feel connected to everything around them.

Figure 1. For energy, clearing the mind, and opening the body. Back should be flat on the floor, tailbone tucked in, upper body relaxed, arms straight up in the air, legs 90 degrees, and flex ankles and wrists. Focus on abdomen, palms and the bottom of your feet for accumulating pure energy, health and vitality.

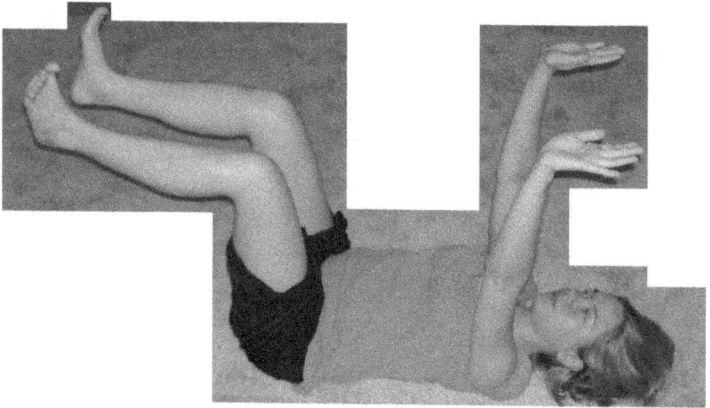

Figure 2. Relaxation breathing pose for stress reduction and calming the mind, focus on inhaling through your nose and feeling the breath fill your abdomen and exhale through your mouth. The pose is ideal for menstrual discomfort, grounding, balancing energy and improving overall health

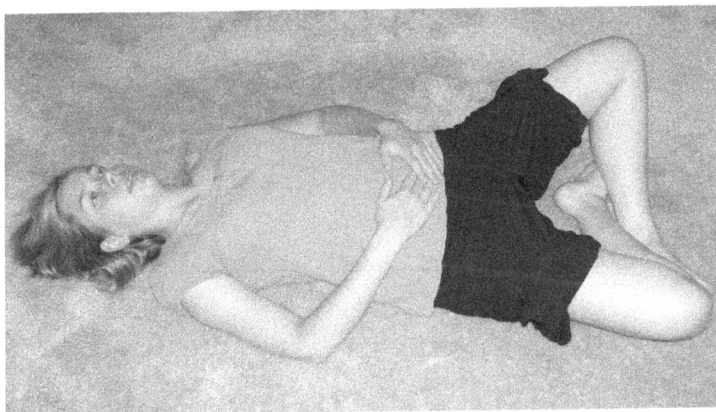

Figure 3. "plow posture" legs behind the head is for energy, stress reduction, focus on the abdomen, relax upper body

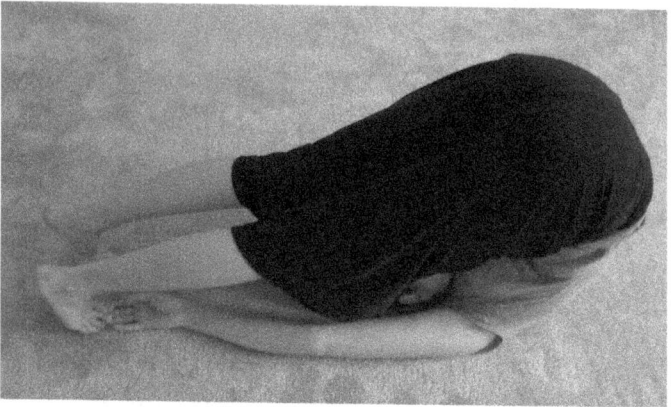

Sheri Gilburth - Licensed Massage Therapist and Reiki Master, Atlanta GA
http://www.heartcentertherapy.com/.

Instruction given by Certified Yoga Instructor Essud Fungcap Jr. Atlanta, GA
http://www.heartcentertherapy.com/.

Qigong

Qigong is a relatively unfamiliar term and practice for many people. It is pronounced "chee gong" and, just like yoga and tai-chi, it is a form of practice that involves refining the body's energy. It is considered a method of developing all systems in the body, especially the nervous system, to have it function at its best. This way the body can heal itself from many potential ailments. This type of practice is advantageous for a single mom since most of what she involves herself in are potentially energy depleting tasks that are only amplified for the simple fact that she may be doing two jobs and playing two roles. My experience with qigong has been a positive one. No practice that can promote circulating, revitalizing, and calming can be negative.

Since I have had some practical experience in tai-chi, I was able to understand that many of these practical exercises are related, down to the original standing posture. It is amazing the effects of something that seems very simple to do, requires one to be still, which many single moms often cannot do. Standing shoulder width apart, with knees slightly bent, erect and clearing your mind initially is not an easy task, but in daily practice it becomes a natural routine. I eventually committed to the six-day routine for two weeks in a row and found that it is very effective in relieving many of my morning aches and pains. I would try fifteen minutes in the morning and fifteen minutes in the evening. This worked better than all of it in the morning because it helped me to sleep soundly. My focus was on relieving myself of the constant feeling of fatigue. It took a while to maintain correct posture to circulate the Qi. It was used also to develop greater intuitiveness and connection to our divine creator. A position I learned is called the *Lying Down Stress Reliever.* The name speaks for itself. I used this most frequently as a meditation exercise since I was able to apply it every night on my bed. Visualizing the negativity leaving was an additive to other nightly routines, such as applying breathing techniques. If you should decide to start practicing Qigong, after some time visit your doctor to get an EEG reading, or find a professional who can offer you information on a bio feedback machine reading to determine stress levels. You may find a difference in levels and you may find yourself motivated to continue adding these techniques to your lifestyle.

Diet & Nutrition

It is necessary to find a healthy alternative consisting of an ideal percentage of calories in carbs, protein, and fat. Even though ultimate health seekers commonly follow a strict regimen, it doesn't mean that the average healthy single mom cannot decrease or increase their percentages a bit to fit their lifestyle, age gender, size, goals, and activity level. As long as the percentages are sufficient so that an individual is on their way to a cleansed body, filled with energy and stamina. Find a practical approach to a low fat diet consisting of a high percentage of good carbs in your diet.

The average American eats only a little less than fifty percent calories from carbs and that much from fat. Even some body builders or athletes prefer to consume all and any foods acquiring a high amount of protein, but know little about the best foods to build muscle and increase energy. Therefore, many diets in America fail the average person and they feel as if they failed themselves. This is why it is important to not only eat the right foods, but to also eat the right proportion of calories in these foods.

For those wishing to maintain a healthy weight, it is best to follow a diet based on Caloronutrients rather than percentage of weight or volume of foods consumed. We are physiologically and anatomically designed to eat certain foods. The simpler the meals the better they are, providing the nutrients our body needs to function at its best. Although, food alone will not make a person healthy, as an individual would need sunshine, water, sleep, rest, fresh air, emotional stability, comfortable temperature, peace and serenity, and physical activity, but imagine sustaining under these elements without the right nutrients to maintain the systems of the body and allowing digestive efficiency. Impaired digestion can lead to constipation, fatigue, gas problems, low energy or sluggish feeling, and irritability. Couple all these with the daily challenges of a single mother's routine and you can rationalize why you feel upset with how life is going regardless of your circumstances.

A man on a three thousand calorie diet can consume the same percentages of calories in carbohydrates as a woman on a twelve hundred calorie diet. Both individuals would have to be careful not to mistakenly confuse the weight of the food for the calories and assume that what they are eating is sufficiently healthy as part of their full day's meal pattern. A small of amount of oil and nuts can account for a large percentage fat in their meal. A modern trend is to load a huge plate of salad with nuts, thinking that since iceberg lettuce may have little nutritional value, they are getting it from the nuts, oils and other "meal enhancing" extras.

It is important to get enough calories for our size and physical activity level so we do not generally under-eat or over-eat fat. A good ratio of calories can help an individual seeking healthier options to set a pace for themselves most conducive to their style of living. This is especially applicable to the single mom since the level of pace and food options can highly impact the level of effectiveness she has on getting things done and achieving her goals.

Furthermore, even if you were not proactively trying to maintain a healthy lifestyle, sooner or later your body will let you know that it is time to do something about how bad you have been feeling and you will suddenly want to inquire about certain exercises such as Pilates or personal training. You may start reading more books about being health conscious, or you may start to meditate or eat healthier. It was Dr. Herbert Shelton, a pioneer in the movement of hygiene who said, "*Primarily, life seeks to preserve itself or rather the organization it has built for itself, "All the functions of life have reference to this effort at self-preservation either of the individual or the race. This is as much true of the single cell as of the complex organism.*" (p12)

There are so many ways to get help. There are so many ways we tell others we don't want or need it. Accepting help is another way of allowing gifts to enter our lives. We meet who we are meant to meet and it is an invitation to connect with someone.

NOTES

Chapter 9
Seeking Professional Help

Many times a single mother may decide that counseling or some sort of therapy could benefit her life. I agree, since her children may benefit as well watching relationships around them improve. Though therapy is always an option for those moms who feel overwhelmed by the stress of single parenthood and tackling unresolved issues, there are other alternatives that may focus more on present and future outcomes. There are also services that help to treat specific areas in a person's life. Some of the services below are meant to treat, but not heal and make no claim of curing. Some are meant to heal and not treat. Some focus on healing past issues and some focus on the present and future only. Some look at physiological aspects or self improvement and others look at changing minor habits. (Please note that only doctors should prescribe medicine). The following describe only some of the mainstream and alternative emotional recovery services available to all parents:

- **Psychotherapy/Mental Health Counseling** *(may also include psychoanalytic, group, cognitive-behavioral, and talk therapies)*
- **E-Therapy-*Providing counseling over the internet via video conferencing, email, online chat etc...(Does not replace traditional therapy)***
- **Psychiatry**
- **Hypnosis/Hypnotherapy**
- **Neuro-Linguistic Programming (NLP) -*alters patterns of thinking for desired results & maintenance of overall well being***

- **Spiritual Counseling**
- **Life & Empowerment Coaching**
- **Nutritional Counseling/Consulting**
- **Reiki/ Chakra Healing/Aura Cleansing/Energy balancing**
- **Health & Wellness Coaching**
- **Business, Organizational & Career Coaching**
- **Mentoring**
- **Naturopathic & Naturorthopathic** *(includes human health by employing the "Hygienic System")*
- **Hair Analysis- Method used to assess nutritional status**
- **Hydrotherapy**
- **Yoga and Tai chi**
- **Acupuncture/ Auricular Therapy** *(enhanced treatment)*
- **Acupressure and Reflexology**
- **Wellness Spas**
- **Qigong (Qi also known as "Chi", life Force & Life Energy)**
- **Other Holistic Therapies such as meridian, crystal etc...**
- **EFT (Emotional Freedom Technique)**

Other therapies such as occupational, physical, and recreational are primarily sought after for physical healing and maintenance, but are still functional in terms of how we can nourish the soul. Art and dance therapy is especially known for its healing effects on the various chakras and simultaneously improves imagination after working on the chakra most affiliated with creativity. You should always do your research to determine the validity and effectiveness of all services prior to using them. It is also recommended to consult with your primary doctor before attempting something you are not familiar with. Second opinions are just as important, but too many may leave you confused. Not all practices are regulated in every state, but it is important to know that whom you are seeing has acquired the proper training suitable to recommend, diagnose, treat, offer therapy, or simply to provide consultations.

NOTES

"Once you make a decision, the universe conspires to make it happen."   Emerson

NOTES

Chapter 10
A Means for the Single Mom

Are you religiously pragmatic? Are you careful in your choices because you are constantly looking for the most practical way to do things? Don't feel alone in this, since just about every single mom I have come across attempts to become a master realist and gave up being idealistic once "reality" hit them. They find themselves doing what is easier, what comes first and what seems most appropriate to everyone else, but puts aside any notion of doing what they themselves would consider to be ideal since it may "send the wrong message to their kids, their family members, and their friends. I mean let's face it, why would a single mom have time to care about things like…Feng Shui right? You would be surprised to learn that one of the most practical things you can do for your home is to bring in as much positive energy to cultivate a loving, functional and productive home environment for you and your kids. Make it your intention to perform the ideal for yourself and your children and life will become a bit easier, thereby making you feel like you have mastered the art of being practical. Things will then seem to suddenly "make sense."

Nonetheless, the single mom has very little time on her hands. There is always a quicker and easier means to an end, but sometimes we just make it harder for ourselves. Here are some ways to make the single parent life just a bit little easier. The following list includes, but is not limited to, ways to simplify life a bit more, while adding a little leisure: (if you haven't thought of them already)

- **Shopping tools (coupon storage book, lists, a list of healthy snacks)**

- **A Computer, Laptop, I-pad, etc... and High Speed Internet (today it's a must)**

- **Cell phone, bluetooth, skype (family plan & other similar devices to enhance communication with the outside world, but be careful not to replace all of your voice and in person conversations with texts and chatting)**

- **Place of residence near public transportation**

- **Feng Shui (Essential for your home life!)**

- **Proper Transportation (It's worth it in the long run)**

- **Reading books (keep books you haven't read yet on the shelf. Don't just stop reading. One day when you WILL have that quiet time, you will pick it up just because and realize it was meant for you to read it at that time)**

- **A Favorite room (if space is limited it could be an area in the house sectioned off just for you, a mini sun-room with a hammock perhaps?)**

- **Candles to enhance mood...just because**

- **Places to socialize where you can mostly be yourself...how about a bookstore café or a lounge with the music genre you like. Don't assume there is none in your area, providing it is safe of course**

- **Banking online or cell phone banking (use cautiously)**

- **Dating online (use extreme caution)**

- **Online Classes (one certification may make the difference in your paycheck & add to your qualifications to enhance your career)**

- **Rearrange your child's room and add color for stimulation**

- **Kitchen (Tip: To encourage yourself to cook more healthy meals, invest in good quality nonstick pots & pans. You will feel like a chef even If you can't cook!)**

- **Fast vegetable slicing/chopping device (Especially for onions. You cry enough don't you think?)**

- **Home décor, aromatic plug-ins, incense, and a pleasant atmosphere (To stimulate the environment. You begin and end with your senses. We hear & see what we don't want to hear & see all day...now use your senses on purpose)**

- Office supplies & equipment such as a an e-fax or fax machine can expedite errands from home while you perform tasks, such as chores

- Triple A *(AAA)* or some automobile program like it (Note: running out of gas mid highway with the kids in the back seat is not an option. Stop making it one!)

- Phone list of *other* (not just your parents) accessible relatives and friends for emergencies (Ask your mom or dad for this. They'll be happy you asked)

- Toys & games you and your child(ren) can share

- Art projects. Try crayons! They can be quite therapeutic

- An appointment calendar on your computer, cell phone or daily planner

- An unobtrusive alarm clock (that doesn't give you the jitters after startling you from your sleep...small changes like that make a difference!)

- Stress reducing and detection equipment (Among many are the Chi Machine: is said to aid in removing toxins by improving oxygen in the cells, increases circulation & improves metabolism, or Bio-Feedback Machine: commonly used to detect stress levels -may be found in some practices)

- **List of resorts to keep in your day planner or on your fridge (Tip: putting souvenirs of your best trips around the home like above your sink while you do the dishes is a great technique & reminder)**

NOTES

Chapter 11
"Terrible Twos" vs. "Terrible Teens"

One of the biggest dilemmas in our culture today is how the pace in which children grow, mirrors what children are made to portray in fictional and reality television. Eight isn't eight anymore and thirteen isn't thirteen anymore. The peculiar fact is that thirteen, thirty years ago, is the thirteen that was appropriate for that time, but may not be appropriate for now. Though, even thirty years ago, there were those who blamed the media for children growing up too fast for their age. To understand this, many parents would determine that the best thing to do is to turn our attention to the present culture in the media and the details of today's socio-economic factors influencing our kids.

"…our "shoulds" may be based more on what we fear may happen then what is happening now, and therefore we cheat our children out of experiences and deprive them of learning more about who they really are."

More research and interest has been poured into the idea of children having attention deficit disorders. We are seeing an increasing number of children demonstrating restlessness in classrooms and at home. According to a lot of adults, this is seen as a bad thing because the restless energy is directed and carried out in a negative way instead of channeled in a positive and proactive manner. We are looking more at how it is demonstrated than what is making the child restless. It is as if the teenager is viewed as a terrible two, simply exhibiting a behavior and not having any reason behind it, other than to get what he or she wants.

Those who are willing to explore reasons a little further are joining a mass of adults declaring that what we are now seeing is an influx of indigo children. Many people believe that these children exhibit one common trait, attention-deficit hyperactivity disorder (ADHD), since what we tend to think as "normal" communication, may be lacking in the indigo child. Though, what they so call "lack" in communication, they make up for in creativity, tapping into their own wisdom, and demonstrating empathy, which in many ways are more effective channels to transmit important messages if the listener desires to evolve spiritually. In other words, we can learn a lot from our kids!

There are a plethora of sites existing today only to call attention to these types of children. Discussing the indigo child in this book would require a lot of space since according to many authors, they have so much to offer the human race and exceed our time. Many times what we adults consider as knowledge and fact, children in general will challenge with wiser words. Consider the following interaction:

"Mommy, can I play outside today?"

*"I don't think so, honey. See that gray cloud
coming in over there? I think it's about to
rain."*
"No, I still see blue skies mommy."

Her child has not seen the gray cloud gradually moving
in from the far left soon to be working its way into the
midst of white puffy clouds and blue sky. The child
only sees what is happening *right now* and desires to
enjoy what is in her view, rather than worry about what
is coming. Why let what may be coming ruin what she
perceives is happening now. To her mother, playing
outside would have meant having to consider a
raincoat, a cloudy and gloomy day, muddy boots, and
slippery sidewalks. Who are we more worried about,
our children or ourselves? If her child isn't worried
about it, more than likely we are thinking about
ourselves. Think about when someone passes on.
After they cross over, we do not grieve for them; we
actually mourn our own loss. The person crossing
over is perfectly happy and healthy. It all boils down to
how we see things. Since children (especially today)
tend to see things differently, they do not react the way
we adults do. This is not to imply that children should
not learn from their parents and grow, as they should.
It is only to imply that our "shoulds" may be based
more on what we fear may happen than what is
happening now, and therefore we cheat our children
out of experiences and deprive them of learning more
about who they really are. Then we wonder why their
attention is short in class and why they are focused on
everything, but what we are saying to them at the
moment. Have you ever noticed more and more of our
children becoming aware of the little things? For
instance, if your child is sitting in the back seat of your
car, is it any wonder to you why, aside from the "are we

there yet" questions, they are noticing and asking about what they see outside? As they grow into their preteens, they start to internalize what they see, as many of them believe they cannot communicate with their parents due to lack of understanding and inability to relate. Nothing has changed, however. Curiosity does not end. They may be curious about other things and communication just differs.

As we grow older we look less at what is in front of us or what is happening in the present, and more at the past and future. Since every individual forms a perspective of what has happened in the past and what is going to happen in the future, the present situation will be unique to everyone. The dilemma is, however, that since children mainly focus on the present, how can we relate to them if we are basing our present decisions on anything, but what's happening now? How can a small child focus on that gray cloud coming in from the left if what she sees in front of her are blue skies and sunshine she can play under and we only focus on the gray one? She becomes impatient and confused. Of course we should always consider a child's safety and well being in our decisions and it is our job to identify the risks involved in their decisions when they are young, but let us re-evaluate our perspectives and perceptions to determine if the situation is doable after setting aside our viewpoint for a minute.

The teen years are not always easy. In fact adolescence is one of the most trying times for parents when it comes to communicating. What is more trying is having to go through these times as a single parent. Having to play two roles, mom and dad, either fulltime or most of the time is not a task many parents sign up for, but it happens. First, consider the possibility that at times we as parents choose to see what we want to see in our children. Because we claim to know our children so well, *since we did raise them*, we are selective in what we consider the level of influence is from the outside world. We claim that the media influences their music preferences and choice of style, but then don't realize how much their friends can influence their beliefs and values resulting in changes in attitude and lifestyle. It is important that we teach our kids to have values, to be an independent thinker and choose beliefs that foster positive and proactive growth. Since training our kids literally starts at home, it is so important that we are trained first. Often times, because single parents undergo so much pressure from all angles, it can be overwhelming to make another decision. We make decisions quickly, based on our own reactions from the past, which nine times out of ten were not so pleasant.

Today many of our teens seem fast-paced, smarter in technology, quick-minded, and more creative. They are met with a world full of new challenges and entered into a new age, where tradition holds less value then individual choice and alternative thinking. Therefore, many of their experiences will be unique to adults living today. In many cases, they are encouraged to be free thinkers out there and then come home to learn to do the opposite. This is not a bad thing, as much as it is counterproductive to the parents. If parents are under the impression that teens are being deprived of important information they should be learning, then they are also going to think they no longer know them, when in fact their teen is someone they choose not to know.

An ideal solution would be to try to understand what they are learning at school and from their peers, and help them to learn how to discern what is appropriate in terms of what works and what doesn't. If you are disciplining only based on religious principles then you realize that your teen has the right to understand the origin of such beliefs. Realize that a spiritual foundation is a channel to what works in life because we are all of spirit. Know the difference between teaching something based on spiritual connection and religious connection. If your teen is joining the football team simply because he needs to belong, rather than because he enjoys it, then maybe football isn't the best route to where he wants to go right now. Helping him to understand that there are other ways to get to where he wants to go rather than say, "Football is a bad choice," he may then decide on his own that the sport isn't working for him as opposed to complaining, "mom wants to rule my life!" Another extra-curricular activity may allow him more of an opportunity to feel connected to others and, simultaneously, bring out his most creative attribute.

NOTES

Relationships can be viewed like a river, going in one direction or a like lake, unmoving, but observed

NOTES

Chapter 12
Relationships

Often times I come across a single mom who claims that that she does not have time for dating, nor the time to "fall in love" with anyone right now. Of course this could be one hundred percent true for that mom or it could be that she is denying herself opportunities for love and romance and using the "no time" excuse because of any or all of the following reasons:

- **She hasn't found the right guy**
- **She hasn't been attracting the right guy**
- **She has not *allowed* herself time to date**
- **She is considering her child's preference (suitable in some occasions, but we will get to that later)**
- **She is holding out for her child's father who may have moved on already**
- **She is comparing every man to the child's father**
- **Her only plan is to date until she is ready to remarry her child's father (meanwhile, he has other plans!)**
- **She has a "sponsoring thought" such as, "single moms only need someone to take care of them."**
- **She is unsociable or deliberately guarded**

- In the midst of a social event she is *ONLY* attentive to her child's needs
- She brings her child(ren) everywhere due to lack of babysitting or untrustworthy childcare
- She uses her job as an excuse to go nowhere
- She has no "energy" to date
- Dating is a waste of time to her so she is only open to "Mr. Marry me tomorrow" leaving her closed-minded to other men
- She assumes most men will reject her after hearing she is a single mom so she cancels or rejects him first
- She is expecting a reoccurring heartbreaking romance like her first one
- She thinks all she would be able to meet are men who are "willing and settling" to date a single mom
- She doesn't want to bother dressing up or finds nothing flattering in her closet
- She wants to prove to the world that she doesn't need a man or anyone for that matter

We tend to forget, just like how happiness is a choice, love is a choice. When we meet someone that presents the potential for us to feel completely happy with it, it also leaves us open for heartache. So, without realizing it, sometimes we choose to be without a partner. A bigger risk is taken by single moms who have dealt with the pain and struggle of, not only a past failed relationship or marriage, but the responsibilities of having to "hold it all together" on her own for her kid(s).

There are certain rules society places on the single mom that she must uphold and maintain if she is to be a "regular" in what I call the "*cultural assembly line*" of life. This implies that if the single mom is to find any romance it must "*seem*" that everything she does in her relationship demonstrates that she has put her child first at all times and in sequential order. If the mom happens to be hanging out at a nightclub with a close girlfriend, in the back of her friend's mind may be holding the following thoughts. First, *has she found a babysitter who would allow her to stay in the club past midnight and not spoil their fun*?

Then, *if she did, is she dressed in the right "party gear" corresponding to my urbane fashion theme to show that we are somewhat "fun" and "available" to meet someone?*

If she meets someone at this club, does this person seem like "life-partner" material and should she waste her time?

Wait, okay this person seems nice, but does he appear to have the money to take her out on a second date?

If they are on their second date, her friend is already wondering if she has told him about her child.

Does this person act like someone suitable to be a father-figure, regardless of sexual orientation? If she likes this person outside her race isn't she worried about cross-cultural differences and conflicts between her child and the new child they could be having together?

Oh yes, people do go that far into the future!

Everyone, including family, friends, cousins, coworkers and neighbors seem more invested in the single mom's future then she or her child are at that moment. Sure, it is common for a true friend to be concerned whether or not her single mom friend of hers is having fun and may even only say, *"I just want you to have fun, that's all."* It is how family and friends may define what "fun" is for a single mom as opposed to how they think it would be for a person without any children. *"Fun"* is often replaced with phrases that include such terms as "at least" or "one day".

"So you don't have a date to the movies, why don't you at least bring your child along?"
Or
"How about one day soon you and I go out, since I'm sure you're unable to attend our group trip next month...it'll be fun."

What would have been fun is if she was invited to go on the group trip in the first place, but it is easy to assume a single mother is not used to that level of fun because of her lack of time to spare, that she would accept any type of amusement and any form of company will do. It is easy to miss that many single mothers and fathers value their time they have without their children as well and would like to spend it the way their friends would normally spend it.

There is one contradiction that deserves repeating, however. Since most single parents do value their time, it is perfectly okay to feel that the best way to spend it is completely alone, without the need to be with anyone, but a TV-remote and some hot cocoa smothered with whipped-cream. The point is that no one can define what you, the single parent, deem as "fun," regardless if it is with twenty friends, or with one special person at a nightclub who seems to not fit your friend's idea of a suitable mate, although, it is not always easy to watch a single mother friend choose a potential horror of a mate. All anyone wants to see is that she is happy, settled and with the right person...for her child that is.

One of the best gifts a single mother can give to her body, mind, and soul, providing that she respects herself first, is to accept the joy of connecting with another person simply because she is not doing some other person's idea of what is "right". No man is an island. You are not somehow robbing your children of happiness by being happy with someone else involved in your life.

You may however, be putting your children at risk if you choose to allow them to witness your dating game, until that someone you feel most confident about comes along. Ned, Fred and Ed do not all need to come for a nightcap in one week and probably even within the next couple of years. Being without one of the parents is not easy for a child. Not only will you probably be confusing your child, causing them to wonder if either of them is potential daddy number two, you may also be exposing your child to a dangerous habit they themselves may adopt later on and feel it is perfectly okay since mommy did it.

When we choose a loving relationship we are opening a door to someone more consistent in our lives, since that someone is more than likely going to stick around if that is how they feel. This is ideal for your child since, besides you, they may not be used to someone "sticking around." Since true love is without conditions and expectations, it is most difficult for the single mother because, the ease required for a single woman who has no child to accommodate such agreements like an "open" relationship does not come easy for the mom, since she has to also think about her child and the risks involved. Therefore, it is important to be honest with a "potential" from the start. This way that special someone is aware of what he is getting involved in. You have a right to ask him to do the same for you.

Without being graphic or volunteering too much information, it is best to be honest with your children about your relationship with your "potential," providing that you mutually understand that this same person could leave tomorrow by choice. Single parents do not have special radars distinguishing the committed from the non-committed. You will not know if the person you have been dating for three years will just up and leave one morning simply because he has had enough of the relationship. We all hope our partner is decent enough to either stick it through or be honest about it. A "potential" who, before meeting you, went through fifteen dates in a month is pretty much a "red flag," but there are those who seem completely consistent from day one and then in six months...poof! They are gone. You really never know. It is up to you to help your child to understand that, although we all learn from each other, someone leaving has usually more to do with them, whether it is how they handled things, their perspective or what they wanted from you, then it does you and your child. The love *you* gave to your mate, however, had more to do with *your* growth and desires than it did your partner at the time because whatever we give to our partners we are attracting back and giving it to ourselves. It boils back down to the law of attraction and it seems to work for many.

If you really help them to understand this, then your "losses" will seem more like necessary divine events you required for your own enlightenment. To a child, it will seem like your partner who left was at a loss and you are at an advantage so to speak, since you will be getting an even better opportunity next time. Believe this and it will happen. It is not easy to come to this while you are actually going through it and I don't recommend convincing yourself of this without going through the grieving process first, otherwise your mind, body, and soul will be telling you different things. If you follow the one that may lead you to a decision your soul knows doesn't work for you, you will be calling that experience to you. Simply be patient with yourself until you're at a peace then you'll be at a better place to make effective decisions. You have to allow yourself to feel sad or emotions will burst out of you when you least expect it, like in the middle of a funny commercial you and your kid are watching together.

Attracting a life partner is like auditioning to be in a commercial or modeling shoot to be headlined in a magazine spread. The judge is not just looking for a pretty face, but also qualities such as, presence, character, originality, confidence, expression of inner strength and beauty etc...You would be surprised to discover how much of these qualities we do and do not display to others when we first walk into a room. You'd also be surprised to know how little we demonstrate these on dates for the fear of the person sitting across the table seeing our true selves and the stories we are attached to.

Your child is a gift and shouldn't be a surprise to your date after the fourth time out together, however do not be so quick to cast out the first "potential" who seems a bit nervous about children, and what I also mean as "potential" is someone who will accept children in his life. If he doesn't have children of his own, most likely your "potential" simply has not been around kids much and has yet to discover his ability and strengths before he builds a relationship with yours.

"Soul Mates"

When we hear most people talk about their "soul mate" they are normally referring to their true love and the end to their search for a partner. Although primary mates exist, we actually have many soul mates, whereas every person we have decided to cross special paths with in our lives are soul mates who agreed to contribute to our experience here on earth. For example, your mother, your child and your old friends are some. Once in a while, however, someone comes across as a "special" person, since they seem to complete each other's sentences, have no expectations, or conditions, feel a sense of "purpose" with, and allows the other person to be exactly who they are. This is a mate who transcends many others and the "life partner" most of us choose.

… Never aim to lose yourself in a relationship, but to know yourself in one instead.

Sometimes you meet someone and things seem to click and this person has yet to come around. At times your "other half" is just not ready. The reason for using the term "other half" for this particular person is because in order for two people to find each other as their true mate, each must be whole or seeking "wholeness" first. You cannot meet someone being a "half" and expect him or her to complete you. Otherwise, the relationship will be a co-dependent one for a long time if it lasts.

Saying, "you complete me" can now mean, "you help me to recognize the parts in me that make me complete" instead, since they are only helping and inspiring you to help yourself towards completion. What would happen if your "other half" went away for a few months? Will you simply fall on the floor and "lose" that part of yourself? Will you not continue to be passionate about the same thing your partner inspired you to feel that way about anymore because he held the "passion key" and went away for a few months? Then as he stays away, you feel something is missing. You believe it is him that is missing, but in actuality it is that part of yourself he brings *out* in you, not *to* you. This is what we mean by "losing" yourself. Never aim to lose yourself in a relationship, but to know yourself in one instead. Let that person be the one who allows you to know yourself more. This applies when people say, "you bring out the best in me!" Not "You're keeping the best part of me. Can I have that key back since you are going away for a while?" This way, that something "missing" will always be accessible for you to work on since it is only something within you, not in someone else.

Sex

At the time when a woman reaches her sexual prime, which is considered to be around her thirties, regardless if she is a mom or not, suddenly dating only once a year doesn't seem to be enough. Since many women have their first child between twenty-five and somewhere in their thirties, hormones are racing, while simultaneously energy seems to be depleting. While boys were peaking earlier, many girls were gearing up for their "life partner." Then when the reality of motherhood hit, mom had to decide if this sudden sex drive was her thorn or her newly discovered weapon. For a woman sexual pleasure has more to do with how comfortable she is with her own body than it does her partner's physical attributes (not ignoring the fact that a partner's performance is definitely a factor).

Have you ever noticed that when you feel most attractive and most confident with how you look and appear to others, you are more willing to give yourself more sensually and freely to your mate in bed regardless of the level of compatibility? Women have actually claimed to have more of a pleasurable sexual experience. Of course the ideal is for two people to be physically compatible, still sexual exchange starts before reaching the bed, especially since for many women it takes a bit more of a romantic effort from the other person before she does the deed.

The challenge moms in general have has less to do with physical capabilities than it does, emotional and spiritual. If a woman's husband left her and their child and then she subsequently had two fast and failed relationships, she may feel the next time she opens herself up to someone she is leaving herself vulnerable and now has to undergo a tough decision process.

If her prime suddenly hits her she may say to herself, *"All I want are casual relationships, no strings attached and on to the next!"* She has to choose if this will benefit her in anyway and if this would fulfill her emotionally and spiritually. Most likely she isn't pondering all this on a conscious level since the body wants what it wants, but down deep inside she knows that the question is whether or not she will feel even lonelier after sex with Mr. One Night Stand number three. Whatever decision is made, it isn't until the single mother taps into what truly makes her feel satisfied, that she will be unaffected by the fact that she may once again be alone after sex. For some single mothers, sex is such a risk to their emotions, that to avoid feeling vulnerable, they just don't even engage in sexual conversations or flirt harmlessly with men.

Feeling aroused and feeling sensual are not quite the same thing. A sexy man doing a "sexy" thing can turn on women, but she exudes sexuality when she feels like the Goddess she actually is and therefore discovers more of her sensual side. Therefore, her best preparation before sex, regardless if it is with her "potential" or with her many one-night stands, is to fuel that fire within.

Some women, no matter who tells them how sexy they are, cannot believe it, at which point she should begin with practical exercises that will increase the female sex drive and her confidence level. If you are medically clear to perform some of these tasks, try the following:

1) Exercises
    a. Sustained jogging (a couple days per week)
    b. Pelvic exercises (kegels)
    c. Abdominal

d. Strengthening Muscles using weights

2) **Look into certain foods such as avocados and dark chocolate to determine the well known effects they have on the libido**

3) **Belly dancing classes or pre-recorded instruction you could play at home...very sexy!**

4) **Sexually enhancing affirmations in front of your mirror. For example:**
   e. "I am so sexy!"
   f. "I am desired!"
   g. "I am confident and excite all my partners."

*note: say it or something similar until you believe it. Then say it again! You will start to see how life around you will support these thoughts. Someone may just come up to you out of the blue and say, "You have a nice smile."

5) **Wear clothes that actually fit! Do all your jeans and shirts fit an extra person? Unless you are violating a cultural standard, showing your shape is good thing, as long as it is tasteful. Check your wardrobe for clothes you never thought to go together in the past. It's a new age!**

6) **Look at yourself in your mirror and attempt to discover other sexy qualities about you and little behaviors you tend to show**
   a) A certain grin that people tend to notice about you
   b) A certain glance you didn't know about before
   c) Your most relaxed state is many times your

sexiest pose. Don't try so hard
d) While saying your affirmations, notice the tone
    and heaviness of your own voice. Be very
    relaxed and then listen to it.

Divorce

The period after a divorce is not often easy for single parents. Depending on the age, it can be doubly as difficult for the child. It is not hard to imagine a parent continuously putting their best face on for their children after the divorce has settled. I didn't say it was to her advantage. I just said it is not hard to imagine. It is counterproductive to pretend that, now since daddy has left, mommy will be the one to fix everything like an independent entrepreneur putting out a fire. It is not a business. He or she is your child.

Separation Agreements are never very easy, but sometimes necessary. Many divorced parents had gone through years past the divorce and had still managed to adhere to a suitable custodial arrangement without an actual separation agreement on file. I would always recommend two people put aside their irreconcilable differences for the best interest of their children, but I would also recommend a conversation discussing the consistency of the arrangement since a child needs some form of structure, especially at an early age. This is important since people react differently to life-altering events and what occurs may impact either custodial parent in a way that suddenly alters parenting skills. Your child's father or "other parent" may have been happy about the divorce, may have been consistent with picking up little Darlene, and then years later her father experiences another divorce. If his reaction is fear-based and he feels completely alone, this may influence his decision to fight for full custody. This can happen the other way around. Mothers are not always the full or even the part time custodial parent. It is often said that it is a challenge for a mother to be away from her child for too long.

A positive approach to revisiting the topic is to simply ask how your child's other parent feels the arrangement has been going. Most people get scared once they feel a question may lead to an accusation or a loss of what or whom they hold dear. So be absolutely genuine and calm while approaching the issue.

I came across a married couple fifteen years ago, who got divorced and never formed an agreement. Both parents were very pleasant and amenable. They were even very friendly towards each other. Then the mother broke up with her boyfriend of two years and suddenly discovered in herself that she desired to have her child. Remember that although court-filed agreements are most effective, it is perfectly fine to document an informal agreement between the two of you so you do not have to go through any legal hassles. Though do not look at legally preparing yourself as an attempt to "stick it to him" or "her," since your child is ultimately affected by this change.

Whether you fall into the upper, lower or middle class income bracket, your child will care least about all the material things he or she may lose or gain; more specifically children preteen and under. Therefore, do not attempt to persuade your child materially, socially, financially and no, not even with food. Do not try to put your child against his other parent by using the idea that you cook more of the food he or she likes, you give an allowance, you have shindigs at your house, or you take him to the best parks. Nothing compares to

having two parents around and all the swaying may bite you back one day causing resentment and bitterness from all ends.

It is not always disappointing if the child is not used to having the other parent around consistently. Some highly evolved children only see happiness and opportunity where we adults see challenges and loneliness. Your child may actually *want* you to find someone new. Don't assume you know exactly what your child desires. Your child may simply be asking for stability in the home, or a bigger family in general, or just for you to be happier then you have been the past few years. It is essential to discuss this with your child, while allowing him to express how he feels about the divorce or separation. Like I said before, a child's one or two phrase feedback could be the very wisdom you need to hear. Trust the process.

Since divorce is so common today, it is exciting to know there are couples out there that have discovered a secret to a long happy marriage. What I truly believe and learned through my own experience is staying together is more about how we treat ourselves so we can be the ideal mate for the other person. Since I am not an attorney, I can only give my opinion, based on my own humanistic values.

You are Not Divorcing Your Child

Remember that the decision to divorce is never an easy one whether it stems from emotional or practical reasons. Nonetheless, it is unhealthy for a child to remain in an abusive, neglectful, or tense environment. So, although divorce is never the ideal, it is better for the child to simply know that both parents will love and continue to be there for them even if mommy and daddy aren't together anymore. When a

child gets used to an environment where they consistently see mom and dad argue and fail to communicate, or treat each other with disrespect, they are at risk in adopting these behaviors in their own relationships as they grow older. A child may grow up only knowing couples can survive this way and will lower personal standards in future relationships simply because this is all they know. Sometimes I come across a dad who expresses that he feels obligated in making up for the neglect he received as a child from his parent and therefore, sacrifices his own wants and needs to stay in an unhealthy marriage for the children. This is a personal choice and sacrificing for the child is noble intention, however think about the oxygen mask in an airplane. If we cannot breathe, we cannot save our children.

Chapter 13
Show *Mom* the Money!

I will not get into all the legalities involved in seeking child support from an uninvolved parent. Since laws for alimony and child support vary in each state and divorced parents are not required to live in the same home, nor the same area, we would require an extensive amount of book space to discuss every scenario leading to the possibility of claiming overdue child support. What you, as the single fulltime parent, can do, however is to start by researching the minimum guidelines to receive child support in your state. This way if or when you are ready to pursue the matter you will be prepared with the minimum the other parent must give or perform to provide for your child and to meet state guidelines.

Alimony and child support are two separate requirements. I recommend that if you have never pursued child support before, do not begin your hunt for both. The needs of the child come first and may come to realize that all those extras going to you could have gone to the child. If you have a job and you are receiving child support at the same time, use *some* of the money you earn at work for your personal need and fulfillment.

Once in a while I come across the single mom who decides that it would not be right to ask for anything outside the minimum child support from the other parent not fully involved in the child's life. The following are some of the common reasons why many single moms hold back from asking:

- She doesn't want to argue with the other parent
- She just doesn't have the time to deal with it

- She feels asking for more is being a little selfish somehow
- She feels since the other parent is doing what he is suppose to do, which is paying the minimum, she doesn't have the right to ask for more
- It isn't the "honorable" thing to do
- Ballet lessons is a luxury and since mom is the one who decided she can take the class, she will just have to pay
- Her belief that a single mother's job is to struggle and show sacrifice, as it builds character
- Down deep she wants to remain the victim
- She would rather rely on the system for financial help **(this is in no way considered a "lazy" choice. The single mom is inundated with many viable options to help her get on her feet for a fresh new start. Parents with certain disabilities may have challenges in transitioning to full independence and may rely on it permanently, but for the average healthy single mother it should only be used temporarily. It would be ideal to work on getting out of the situation requiring you to depend on government assistance. If you continue to do absolutely nothing, but accept assistance then you *are* really just taking the "easy way out")**

It took the two of you to conceive a child and it usually takes a village to raise one. Raising children is not a part time commitment; no matter how many evenings you hire a babysitter. You are raising your child while you are at work, while you are dining out with friends, even while you are in the bathroom because you are

not suddenly going to stop being concerned for Joey Jr's well being at any moment during the day. These days, the role of "mom and dad" have taken on new meaning, since same sex marriages have been legalized in some places, but for the sake of making a point for the single mom, let's use the "father" as the non-custodial parent. Taking two hours for yourself does not mean that you are not being a parent during that time. Unfortunately, the father may argue on behalf of himself since you two have agreed you would have your child most of the time. The risk he is taking, however is relinquishing his right to be part of the major decisions you have to make for the child you share. He is also giving up the opportunity to witness or immediately become aware of some of the more important milestones in his child's life. This may not matter to him now, but it may surprise him to realize one day that he actually wants to know what his kid is up to and how his child has resolved certain issues you made him aware of in the past.

Children do not stop at Christmas, and birthdays when it comes to asking for something they want. Moms do not stop at fieldtrip fees and lunch money and do not stop at dance classes and karate lessons when it comes to dishing out the funds. Let's show mom the money for the *other* moments in her child's life:

Some of the "Requests" Commonly made by Kids

"Mommy, can we stop over there? I'm hungry. " (You both just left the house after you've just made pancakes and eggs for both you & your child)

●

"Mom! I dropped my toothbrush down the toilet again. I'm going to need another one for tonight!"(At any age)

●

"Mom I know I'm sick, but do you have to buy me that yucky medicine today?" (The Toddlers, Pre-Kers, the grade-schoolers)

●

"Mom, I know you may have probably wanted to know this before we got here, but I sort of owe the library twenty-five dollars for overdue books and it has to be paid before you could check anything out. Thanks for understanding!" (If they are old enough to check out a book on their own, they are old enough to earn the money back to pay for it)

●

"Mom, it's valentine's day. Can I have some money to get flowers, candy, chocolates, this heart-shaped pendant, a teddy-gram online and a bracelet for my new girlfriend?" (A teenager not old enough to work)

●

"Mom can I borrow fifty bucks? I broke the neighbor's vase again." (A hyper twelve year old boy perhaps?)

●

"Oh yeah, I forgot to give you this permission slip due last week. The tickets need to be paid for tomorrow. I'm the club president. They're counting on me!" (You can teach her that if she were trying to demonstrate reliable leadership skills she should have been responsible enough to give you the slip two weeks ago, but now you have to decide if teaching her this lesson is worth her losing the opportunity to be part of something she enjoys.)

●

"Mommy, I just clicked a "Use Pay-pal" button on the computer and it said 'thank you for your contribution.' What does that mean?" (Have parental control over that computer mom!)

Those unexpected expenses are just that...unexpected, and uninvited. Therefore, it will only hurt you to hold back from informing the other parent of these small, but many expenses. If this is your first child with him then it is quite possible that he may be unaware that children tend to require, demand, or desire more and more as they grow. The items may be smaller than a Tonka toy truck, but I am sure you would prefer paying for an over-sized toy over a mini touch-screen cell phone any day. The child's other parent may also be ignoring it and is not rushing to pay since you are not bringing it up.

There was no handbook for you and your partner to read before deciding to have a child. In fact many people who even believe that child raising is costly, still did not anticipate the "extras" needed on a day-to-day basis. Therefore, it is not unreasonable to expect a little extra support for your child since day care, at least, will cost you a few hundred dollars per month for one child alone. Do not make excuses simply because you feel bad, you feel God will punish you for asking, you want to look like the good guy or you want to remain appearing like the victim. None of it serves a purpose other than to attract harder lessons down the road. No one is "schooling" you but yourself regarding this issue.

You are also meeting your needs by working to make life a little bit easier than you have been making it. It is mainly your child's wants and needs that the other parent may not know comes up once in a while. What you are demonstrating to the other parent is that, although *you* are trying to provide a leveled playing field for your child to have fair chances, it is not completely even if you are *willingly* cheating his child out of opportunities. Some children, even with both parents living with them, are forced to live without items many middle and upper class families would call "just another school supply" or "just another toy." So to willingly deprive a child simply because mom and dad are bitter after the divorce, will serve no one.

Mom may also want to start saving for her child's college tuition. This is another decision she may be making independently. It is her right to decide when she feels is the right time to open this account. You may decide that your retirement fund will cover the tuition when the time comes, but is it fair to use what is ultimately intended for your "retirement" when the responsibility is on both of you? If the child's other parent is not around at all, then you have to do what you have to do, but until then it doesn't hurt to make the other parent see how a little extra goes a long way.

Living Paycheck to Paycheck

These days, it is not only the single mom who finds herself using her entire paycheck to pay bills. Whether it is the gas bill or daycare tuition, it seems that mothers, in general, are tightening their purse strings. At the end of the day however, the current economic state has very little to do with spending habits when it comes to how you treat yourself. Some of the money has to go to something you can afford to do and purchase for yourself. That is, if you break your check down into percentages as opposed to choosing a random amount to spend, which of course would be shopping on impulse. I also said "do" because some people feel that doing something like donating money to a charity is like doing something for themselves.

If you are into zodiac signs, they say Libras are impulse shoppers. Being a Libra myself, I can understand the desire for beautiful things, but just like a toddler needs to control grabbing things he does not need at that time, we would do best to control ourselves from buying stuff we don't immediately require as well. You can see a financial consultant or seek the advice from a friend who seems really diligent with her savings and has good credit, but seek different opinions. Friends may be good at saving, but if they are not using some of it to repair their credit it may not do any good to seek advice from them about how and where to obtain a loan with a low interest rate. Of course this is considering that you live in the United States, where the issue of credit has become one of the country's biggest quandaries.

Unless you feel you absolutely have no choice, try to spend a small percentage on yourself every other week after you have received your paycheck. If you receive your check weekly you can choose to spend that percentage each time, but it is more common to feel guilty pampering yourself weekly, as opposed to bi-weekly when it seems like you have given yourself enough time to come down from your shopping "high." I generally recommend ten percent of your biweekly amount (weekly amount if you have the control). If you spend ten percent, no one can ever say that you do not do anything for yourself.

Here is a simple breakdown that may work for you:

1. Get paid: $800.00 every two weeks

2. Spend $80.00 on something you like such as an outfit, jewelry, music and DVDs, an interactive software game, dinner, movies, dancing etc...

3. You have $720 to pay for the minimum you owe on credit cards and bills.

This is in no way an attempt to get you not to pay your bills. You should always pay your bills, though consider this: If you decided to use your last $80 on the remaining credit card bill you have not paid yet then bear in mind how much of that is actually reducing your balance until the next bill arrives. If the next bill shows an amount that seems very close to what it was before you paid the $80 then you are left feeling as if your money could have been better spent treating yourself to a dinner out with friends or your family.

According to the *U.S. Department of Labor's Bureau Labor of Statistics (BLS)* survey in (2009), the average U.S. consumer spends their annual paycheck on the following:

Transportation................................$7,658
Food...$6,372
Housing..$16,895
Tobacco and smoking supplies............$380
Insurance and Pensions $5,471

Entertainment...................................$2,693
Alcoholic Beverages............................$435
Cash Contributions...............................$1,723
Reading..$110
Healthcare..$3,126
Education..$1,068
Personal Care Products and Services....$596
Apparel and Services...........................$1,725
Miscellaneous $816

Besides tobacco and alcohol, the average American consumer spends the least on reading, contributions, education, and personal care and service. Is it any wonder why we seek alternative ways to get results in life? Is it any wonder, after paying so much for the house, transportation, food, clothes and daycare for our kids, medical bills and insurance, we are not seeking refuge in spirituality, self-healing and tasks requiring the use of our imagination? If the above list demonstrates similar spending habits then take some time to consider what your priorities are and where you would like to allocate your money for the long term, but remember to save some of it for you to enjoy your *now* moments.

We often use our paycheck to pay the minimum of many credit cards and then in the same week use all the same cards up to their spending limits. Sometimes we get fed up with one overbearing creditor who will just not stop calling and out of impulse you almost use your entire paycheck to settle the account. I don't suggest doing this unless you have extra funds placed on the side or have come into a large sum of money suddenly, when you could simply pay all of them off. Though it is good to pay off what you owe and have a balance of zero, it looks even better to show consistent payment history overtime. Therefore, try to develop a payment regimen using your paycheck that you receive from your job. You can also ask the bank to open up an account you will only pay bills with. With online bill paying or automatic bill pay, it has become easier to budget our wallets and our time. Please be cautious before attempting to use anything fast and easy. The fast and easy method you use to put money in your account could be the fastest and easiest way for someone else to take money out.

The key to success is Balance.

NOTES

Chapter 14
Balancing Priorities

To juggle between what your child needs from you, what your boss requires of your work, what your family insists on seeing, and what your lover wants from your time and energy, demands a level of focus that requires a different sort of strength. In other words, you are required to wear a different hat at different hours of the day and start all over tomorrow. Then you must do all of this looking good too! Let's face it we mothers really try to do it all! We attempt to declare how independent we are by being what everyone feels we should strive to be, whether it is strong, courageous, inspiring, energetic, or desirable. For some of us our level of independence *depended* on what everyone else wanted us to do. Does that make sense?

This is what we call going for the single mom of the year award and trying to show that we can manage without anything or anyone else since we have already proven we can raise a child alone. Of course, there are those who are willing to remain in a victim, "woe is me," status, but there are those who are reaching the other end of the spectrum by trying to overachieve amongst the overachievers.

Overachieving

When I received news I was accepted for a program I applied for to further my education, I was inspired and had also determined that I might as well do everything else too! I thought, I should start my third book, work full time, sing more songs at church, start a youth choir, get more clients using a new marketing technique, and be super mom all to start my new trend! After a couple of months I realized the only reason I wanted to do it all was because I held the idea in my mind that one great achievement was a sign for me to get the ball rolling on some other milestones. I had begun to feel overwhelmed and I hadn't even started the tasks yet. I then realized I failed to follow what I knew down deep, and that is to strive for balance. We should carefully choose tasks that will not burn us out in one area of our lives so that we neglect another.

What many single moms tend to forget is that the ultimate achievement is to acquire a lifestyle that enables them to balance all parts of who they are and what they do. We have touched on overachieving earlier in this book, but the topic of balance deserves further elaboration, since to achieve it, should be a significant goal.

Balancing Relationships with Yourself

Let us take, for example, a single mother whose life is not devoted completely to her lover or partner. All the effort and energy it takes to please him will be exhausted the moment she feels she has not received what she desired in return. She may fight and fight for his attention and the more she tries, the less he wants it. When you are more and more engrossed in the affairs of another, whether you are doing it with good intentions or not, you are devoting time you need to develop yourself to become who your mate was attracted to in the first place. It is essential to have a balance between the energy you offer in your love life and the energy you offer yourself. The ironic thing is that the more you work on yourself, the more you are offering to your partner then if you were to try so hard while simultaneously neglecting your needs.

A point to remember is that there are those partners, who no matter what you do or don't do, it is neither, ever enough or it is too much. This is when you have met someone you will probably end up growing out of. You are with him to learn what you need to learn in order to grow. When they continue to be dissatisfied they have not reached your level of growth and will continue to remain stagnant. In this case, try to move on to someone you will not have to "carry" for the rest of your life, who will inspire and help to build you up. Aside from these cases, it is a great benefit to you to balance your life with doing something you are passionate about. If you are busy doing this, your down time will not be spent worrying about what your partner is doing, but rather what you would like to do for yourself or what you love. This is good self-preparation for marriage. We women spend so much time planning for and preparing our future wedding and spend less time on preparing ourselves for the actual marriage.

I found that several of my clients come with the idea that to fix a marriage there is something or someone, other than themselves, they need to address first. Since we cannot control what others do, we can change the way we see things by changing ourselves, thereby changing the ultimate outcome of the situation. One action does lead to another.

Another scenario would be if you spent all of your time and energy on a partner, that you neglect the needs of your child. We are not talking about outright abuse. Most moms I meet do their best to provide at least the bare necessities to their child. I am referring to the need for your *quality* time, not just your time. Balancing love with a partner and quality time with your child can pose as a challenge if they have not yet formed a close relationship and you are challenged with the need and desire to share yourself with both. When you achieve balance in the many areas in your life you find a middle ground to everything and actually enjoy your experiences rather then perceiving the actions as "stretching yourself thin." It is imperative that you do not take for granted the time you have with your children since they are only young once and your adult partner is remaining an adult from now on. So if you really had to choose then decide to establish a routine break from everything else so this space is filled with quality time with your child. Your child will depend on this space and time, and your days will be a bit more structured.

An unbalanced approach would be to promise your children they will have all of your attention everyday this week from morning to night simply because you feel so bad that you were too busy last week. What will end up happening is that at the end of this week you would have missed or neglected something you really wanted or needed to accomplish, but put aside. Then it will return ten-fold. For example, let's say you decide that your eleven-year old daughter needs your attention this week so that you and she can complete a science fair project together. This is perfectly acceptable since it the project that needs to get done and she is simply asking for your help. Though, imagine that you decided to use this time as "you and her time" only. Your partner calls on Wednesday to confirm plans you made last month, but you forgot since you are concentrating on the project only. You have a work deadline due in two weeks, but decide to put it off since this week is strictly off limits. You miss a few calls from your friends because you know you can return them on Saturday and you decide to order pizza and eat quick pre-packaged meals all week so that you can still enjoy the time you are spending on this project. Then Sunday rolls around and you realize that you forgot to return most of your friends' calls. You find yourself having a heart to heart conversation with your partner because he feels you are suddenly avoiding having to meet that date you discussed happening in the future. You feel you have no energy for him anyway because you ate poorly all week and did not squeeze in time for healthy meals, and your pre-teen actually wants some space from you since you overflowed her with your maternal presence. In this case you are not going to be spending time like that with your pre-teen anytime in the near future and you have missed the opportunity to teach her how to demand your time in a balanced way. Since moms also want a life, you want to set a standard for yourself from the beginning.

You do not want anyone to get used to you giving way too much of yourself because when you are ready to pull back, they are either very upset and angry with your abrupt departure or they cannot seem to get rid of you fast enough. Either way there is no middle reaction in this and therefore you don't feel that things are balanced like you tried to make them. An unbalanced lifestyle has a way of creating a domino effect of problems. Since you are overachieving in one area and neglecting another, somehow what you neglected catches up to you like an avalanche and what you overachieved in leaves you feeling like you are missing something.

NOTES

Be Grateful to those who help to bring out the best
version of you.

NOTES

Chapter 15
Life Coaching for the Single Mom

Life Coaching has been a growing trend and will continue to grow as long as it is successful. Since Coaching has proven to help people succeed, I don't see the trend dissolving any time soon. What gives the industry a good name in my opinion is the idea of helping the client cut right to the chase in where they want to be in life and designing a plan to help them get there, whether they are long or short term goals. Not every coach uses the same approach, but I would say most out there know that the idea is to help an individual to see the results they wish to see. A coach may even help a client discover that the intended path is ultimately not the path they truly desire. This is not always identified through therapy, but many times through the actual tasks the client are motivated and encouraged to perform. This is why, with or without a life coach, it is important to try new experiences. If you do not take risk sometimes, you will find that your fear has prevented you from attracting opportunities aligned with your true purpose and desires.

In terms of how life coaching can benefit a single mother, it is an even bigger and more exciting trend. Often times single parents in general get lost in the "appropriateness" of parenting, they find themselves unable to find loopholes that allow them opportunities that married couples with children have. For example, a married couple with two children may establish a routine schedule that allows them time to do what they love. A Husband and father may spend his Sundays or Mondays playing gulf, dominoes, or watching the game with his buddies and the wife and mother may spend her Saturday afternoons at the salon or shopping with her other married or unmarried friends (most likely married). They have discussed and agreed on this schedule and have made it so it doesn't interfere with their time with the kids.

For a single parent, if they do not have the luxury of available and affordable childcare, designing a plan for their leisure activities and seeing it as an ongoing routine seems pointless at times. Since many single parents encounter unpredictable schedules, they can only design a plan for the short term, as they feel it may only last that long. This does not have to be the case, however. There is no rule out there that states that single parents cannot designate time for fun and leisure, relaxation, and health promoting activities, projects and community service, and more.

For this reason alone, the single parent could benefit from coaching. The time they may put aside for therapy or counseling they could use to actually perform tasks that get them to where they want to be. Don't get me wrong, therapy and counseling have proven to be very successful in its attempt to help a client resolve issues and move past emotions related to past trauma, but a client may be more inclined to work with a coach for that extra push; less talking and more doing; less reflecting on the past and more motivation or inspiration for the future. Since it takes full commitment of the client for coaching to actually work, it will take a leap of faith and a change in perception of how a single parent feels their time should be spent. Should their time be spent mostly worrying if whether or not they will ever live out their dreams or should it be spent working towards that dream? I am hoping it's towards.

For many people, whether single, married, childless or parents, it actually takes getting out of that train of thought that makes them believe simply sitting and wishing is easier and, therefore, somehow a productive use of their time. Nothing is done to reach their goals and they remain the victim, as if we could actually be one. There is no such thing as a victim in life. Yes, of course there are cruel acts beyond our beliefs that people will and have attempted to inflict on some of us. It is difficult to comprehend the motive behind physically or emotionally abusing anyone on purpose, but even from the time of getting up in the morning, we have chosen our actions. We have chosen to be at certain places at certain times and we have also chosen to ignore divine guidance that leads us to better choices. We are also presented with opportunities all day that allow us to choose between this and that, and when we choose that, we end up at an unfortunate place that makes us believe we are victims of bad luck.

When we take the responsibility out of someone else's hands we can better control the situation. This pertains to many incidences in life. Let us look at a metaphor involving a box in front of you. If you look at the box you can remove it out of your way, but if you deny its existence and walk right past it the box will still be there. All you did was ignore it. Use this analogy when it comes to what you see as problematic. Many pain management professionals use this approach to help a client self-heal. Even though the professional is helping, your mind is really doing all the work. This is exactly what a coach is there for, to help by empowering, guiding, motivating, identifying what doesn't work and helping you to see what does. There is someone behind you all the way, but you take the initiative to begin.

Women in general are communicators. Single mothers, regardless of how independent she is or wants to be will eventually communicate with someone about her anticipated plans or lack there of. Since she is a communicator, she more than a single dad may seek out someone who will simply listen. Then at that point, a coach's job will be to motivate her to go further then what she has so-far imagined. A single dad may not communicate as much, but since to many of them plans are not just about talking them through, but rather doing to see results, then the coach *is* the ideal approach. A coach focuses more on the present situation and future goals. Since many single parents put the idea of major achievements so far in the future, if even at all, until their child grows independent, it is advantageous for them to seek alternatives to help them find their true potential.

About Getting Results

I think we can agree that most people desire to see results manifest in their lives. Usually we think of what we want and that thought is followed by how fast we want it to appear. Normally, a client going to a coach because they want to see results in a certain area is not asking for something they see happening twenty years from now. Just as in exercising to lose weight, many people become anxious when they have stopped seeing results or they have hit a plateau. They feel nothing they are doing is producing what would normally happen for some other individual and start comparing their pace, how they are doing things, and what they look like when they are doing it. This is all because we have standards not based on our own spiritual, physical, and mental growth, but someone else's. This is perfectly normal and quite common, but often times meet with someone or something that reminds us that it is not the exercise program, nor any other external factors. It is our beliefs and the view of our own potential. *We* aren't moving with all the externalities that are invented to help you see results.

People are not always aware of why they aren't succeeding in getting results somewhere, but a good determination would be to identify another priority you are neglecting and see if it is affecting your results in this particular problem. For example, if you seem to be repeatedly failing an exam to certify you or license you for something, and you know you have done nothing with your time but study over the past several months you could be unaware that the little time you spent on balancing your time with fun, healthy activities, rest is what contributed to your lack of concentration and, therefore not passing the exam. Being unaware of all that you deprived yourself of is, in itself, a deficiency in your path to balance. We tend to deny that we have not been giving ourselves other things that we need because we are so focused on one over-achieving in one personal area of growth. It is normal to get excited about acing the exam, but isn't the whole point to actually pass it? The result of "passing the exam" is pointless when the process in which you partake in is lacking what is necessary to get you results. Even if you fail, the process you went through was never a mistake since now you can simply learn from it and do it differently the next time. It is when you learn from this that your accomplishments are met sooner. This is what is meant by "making life a little bit easier" than how we have made it. We will go through something over and over again until we get it right.

NOTES

"If there is anything that we wish to change in the child, we should first examine it and see whether it is not something that could better be changed in ourselves."
Carl Jung

NOTES

Chapter 16
Honor Your Child

More and more today women are accepting the life of single motherhood with no regrets and with plenty of pride. The reason for this is values are changing and women are becoming more independent and confident of their own skills. Moms are encouraged to go back to school to learn a new skill or enhance their current one. More fathers are accepting of this and are agreeable. Some are even willing to help. This levels the playing field for moms a bit more and soon, statements like, *"I'm a single mom...I can't"* will fade along with yesterday's catch phrase and become just another cliché. With the increase in single mom's finding who they really are and discovering new talent and independence, it seems appropriate to see our children as individuals and gifts, as opposed to just responsibilities" and little people coming in between you and having a life.

We do not own our children. We are honored with the chance to be chosen as their parents. Since we do not own them, we have to allow them opportunities and give them room to make "mistakes." We do this while we teach them the fundamentals to survive, consistency for that sense of security, and also the wisdom to feel free to pursue what they are passionate about. Of course children will grow up and do certain things that will make us wonder if we were good parents. All parents experience this at least a few times, while their children are alive and kicking. We cannot blame ourselves for every "mistake" they make, as they too must find their own way, while we get out of it.

Honor Yourself

If a single mom can remember to honor her own soul, do what she is passionate about and seek to know who she is, she will discover that there is not a lot keeping her from success and happiness like she assumed during her initial stages of motherhood. The journey begins with throwing away all misconceptions about what our thoughts are based on: our own fears and someone else's opinion of how single moms should live their lives.

To accomplish what you desire you must change your thoughts about how you perceive a result and the outcome will somehow work for you whether you see it immediately or eventually. *However, there is always a way to see results a lot faster!* Once you start altering your thoughts, start reaching for a positive feeling to align with your those thoughts, and replace the word "struggle" with "steps" or "speed-bumps," you will start to see the universe support what you perceive your journey to be, a smoother ride. The universe can only respond to how we perceive a situation to be, offering the gift of ultimate control of our own destiny. Of course, every person has a predestined path, but we have a choice to take the easy way, the hard way, or take a different route altogether. Though, remember that if you have a greater calling, no matter what your line of work is, you will always feel something missing until you get there. Why not arrive at your destination quickly by choosing to use what you have learned from an experience to your benefit.

I realized it is hard to accept that the children we raise solo offer us numerous opportunities for greatness, growth, and enlightenment. It is because our divine creator fortunately allowed us to create our own chances to grow spiritually and experience happiness the way *we* choose, that we think we are continuously punished for our choices. If we are offered free will to make choices and all we need to do is recognize this then, why would we be punished for it? Whether you are a single mother raising a very challenging child or a single person raising a very challenging partner, you would benefit from remembering that you attract your own experiences you learn how to get out of or to alter them to your advantage. Since you are inundated with decisions, why not seek that place that allows you to make better, more productive ones so that both you and your child win in any situation, together.

Single parenthood is an unmatched experience. However, all of the assumptions and various stigmas that go with the journey prevent many single moms from really experiencing it as beneficially life altering and positive. In the past we only used to say, *"It must be tough being a single mom."* With so many resources now we may say, *"It must be tough for that single mom to not have landed that executive promotion this year."* What the single mom wants to hear is, *"I knew she (the single mom) would get the job, she is good at meeting her deadlines."* If she is good at her job, then the idea that she is a single mom is irrelevant, unless it consistently interferes with her work.

The trend, or rather *common belief* has often been that in order for single moms to have a life, they must wait until a child grows significantly independent of their mothers. Then single mothers get jaded, thereby impacting their lifestyle, reducing healthy diets, eliminating healthy attitudes, coping skills and decreasing exercise. "I'm a single mother" is mentioned more as a taboo than a fact. It may seem more of a risk to a single mom to think outside the box or independently than most since many are solely responsible for how the child turns out. All eyes are on mom. For example, an individual may see a female co-worker in the rain rushing for a cab, then she drops her coffee and umbrella, appears annoyed, and is cursing at the driver for splashing water on her after speeding to a halt, some of us may automatically think, "She has it rough! Must be tough to handle making it to work everyday and raising a child alone at the same time. I feel bad for her kid too. He probably barely sees her." When in fact her child has been at his grandmothers, the driver was commonly impatient when he drove, and she spilled her coffee because she tripped. All this did not occur because she is a single mother.

You Too Have a Purpose

It is creative to think independently because the thought comes from you originally. When you are creative, and can use it, you feel more alive and that you are living with purpose. We tend to discover our purpose while we are creating. In fact being the person your child sees the most (other than teachers), you will probably adopt more imaginative and creative projects at work. Children have a way of rubbing off on us in a positive and more productive way. Your purpose is reflected in all you do however, through building relationships, building projects, and building a lifestyle. A single mom may date a man for only a month only to learn he had a month to live. Prior to his passing he resolved many of his own issues through knowing the struggles of the person he was dating. Purpose could reveal itself in our lives while we are creating an open and receptive environment with others where we can exchange information without fear and manipulation.

Assuming a role everyone else feels you should play impedes on your overall growth, creativity, and individuality so that seeking professional help or aid from friends accomplishes nothing if mom is not willing to release those beliefs holding her back from living the life she desires.   How the single mom perceives her journey is key to accomplishing what she desires to be, do, and have and it is many times through her children she comes to realize this.

Sunny Fungcap

Questions And Answers

Sunny Fungcap

Q: What is the best way to spring the news to my parents that I am going to have a child alone?

A. There is no better way to tell your parents, then to just tell them straight. If your parents are supportive, they will have to accept the news and help you to find resources to help you through this new chapter in your life. Accept the fact they may express some disgruntled feelings towards you, but you are still getting the support nonetheless. At least it shows a form of caring. If they are not supportive of your decision to raise a child without a father, providing that you have done what you could to allow your child's father to get involved, it is you that will be living with your decision, so whether or not they are pleased, announcing the truth will leave you less to deal with later.

Q. I am currently taking dance classes at night while my mother watches my kid. Does this seem selfish? Should I be going to school instead?

A. I cannot tell you what you should be doing with your life. I can only tell you that if a dancer is what you ultimately want to be then it will be the reality that you manifest it to be. There are tons of single moms who dance fulltime. Though, unless you are already professionally dancing, I urge you to research all the ways you can seek financial security in this field. I often advise people to identify at least two industries they can see themselves in and get educated, licensed, or certified in it so you can fall back on one if the other is not for you. Remember, EVERYTHING is a choice.

Q. My parents are very disappointed that I will not allow my child's father in his life. He will be born with no father. I made this decision because the father is not ready and is into hobbies not safe for the baby. Am I doing the right thing?

A. If the child's father poses a threat in any way to the child then you have every right to feel concerned and distant, but make sure you are not assuming that the father has not decided to make some changes with himself because he knows he will be a father. Whatever pace and steps a man takes, it may have taken learning the news of him being a father to come correct. Do your parents know what he does that makes him a threat? If they do and they are upset with you without a smidgen of empathy for how frightened you must be then at this point your child may not be in the forefront of their minds. They may be thinking more about you being alone and unmarried.

Q. I really feel like I have permission to do the things I enjoy now, but why do I need permission?

A. That's the thing. You don't! I am going to assume you are over eighteen. We now live in a world full of resources for almost every kind of challenge...well what we may consider challenges anyway. You never needed permission. Maybe you needed to know others may be feeling what you are feeling and that a single mom reaching all her goals is not unheard of!

Q. My sister is sixteen and pregnant. I am nineteen and in my second year in college. My mom is helping her at home and the father is young and not involved. I don't mean to sound selfish, but I fear that suddenly I will have all this responsibility as an Aunt when I am still undecided with what I want to do with my life. How should I handle this?

A. I understand your agitation about the fact that your teenage sister became pregnant so soon, however I am a bit concerned that you are so worried about how much your life will be interfered with when your sister is at home overwhelmed with very difficult decisions, such as how will she finish school and when? She is probably dealing with self-esteem issues, which is common for a teen even without a child. She may feel that her dating life has ended already, and that her dreams are dead (which they aren't of course). You have lots of time to carry on with your dreams, but very little time to spend with your baby niece or nephew. Try balancing out the time you spend working on your goals and the time you spend helping your sister through this. That doesn't require much time and a phone call isn't too much. This could very well be you. It is a double positive to help your self and another at the same time.

Q. I am a single mom and I look good! The issue is that my friends can dress trendy when we go out. When I do the same it seems to imply that I am not doing the responsible thing.

A. Excuse my sarcasm, but are we in the sixties? As long as it is tasteful and your attire spells "lady" and not…well, something else, it is perfectly okay to dress the way your friends do. I am assuming you don't mean wearing *exactly* the same dress. In that case one of you does need to take that off. All kidding aside, you were a lady who liked to have fun before you became a mom and you are the same lady now. The only difference is that you probably need to structure your time more than your friends do and you probably may not own as many of these outfits since your money is budgeted differently. I am so happy you acknowledge the beauty that is you! Dress it up if you want to.

*Note: Sometimes it is difficult to know how to dress to go out without worrying about sending the wrong message to your child. Especially in regards to our daughters, we worry that when they start to dress a certain way we don't necessarily approve of, that we maybe had something to do with it, whether it was because of the way *we* dress, or how lenient or strict we were. The goal is to teach your children the value of their bodies, how not to be afraid of being an individual, and the importance of respecting themselves. This may not always come across, but if you consistently try, you may find that your child will decide more appropriately on their own.

Q. I have three kids. How do I find time for prayer and meditation?

A. Even though it is a good practice to set aside some time each day to do this, it can be just as effective to you if you did it at anytime during the day, while performing some other task. For example, if you want to pray, while you cook, have that conversation and conclude with giving thanks for another well spent day, being alive and happy, and being blessed with that child of yours. The universe works with your intention behind your actions. So even if you meditate, while vacuuming, you are influencing energy. Though, I wouldn't suggest meditating while you vacuum. You may run into your cat.

Q. I am thirty-five and a single dad. Do you think it is too late for me to go back to school?

A. I am glad dad wrote! Absolutely not! Now, more than ever, people are going back to school to discover new careers, even after leaving an old one. In fact, I know people who have been laid off and have suddenly started a business or went to receive further training in something else. Recognize that we all have chapters in our lives. Some, we've left behind were hard lessons and traumatic experiences. We've all had our share. I, myself, am still learning as a mom and a woman. We don't always stay with the same people, the same jobs, or even the same hairstyle! That right there should tell you that each journey is about discovering another part of you or an opportunity to reinvent yourself. Unless you are physically or mentally incapable, it is never too late to start something new. Where is the rulebook that states otherwise? When was the meeting that announced that we must do the same thing forever and at all times? I didn't get that memo.

Q. I am twenty-nine and am interested in recapturing what I had with my baby's father. What should I do, if he isn't responding?

A. Am I to understand that you want to recapture what you had with your baby's father, or do you want to recapture what you had with your baby's father, with someone else? If you want to resume what you had with the baby's father, then first make sure that your love for him is not unrequited. If it is then, all you could do is focus on you and the child and allow time for him to care for his boy or girl. Do not play games. Do not use the child in any way to get him back. Do not pretend you are more helpless than you actually are, and do not prevent him from dating others *if he is now single* by calling his women and letting them know you are the only true love in his life since you have a child with him. If you both want it and you desire an improved relationship with him this time, you have to have grown and learn from why you broke up in the first place. Let it be a natural process so that both of you becoming a family again turns out to be a genuine experience. If you are speaking of recapturing this with another man, then do not seek to "recapture" the same thing. Seek to *capture* a new experience with this new person. New and original is what attracts you to each other. You shouldn't like someone because he is like your ex. You should like him for who he is. He may have similar qualities, but may choose to express these qualities differently in response to *your* level of growth and development.

Q. My boyfriend and I would like to move in together, but he is not that close to my kids yet. Do you think it is the right time for this move? I don't want to force their relationship, but he and I are eager to move forward with this.

A. I understand your eagerness. Love is love, however the issue is not simply that the kids and your boyfriend aren't cozy yet, thereby running the risk of constant friction in the house between them. You have to realize that their relationship will affect how you function as new roommates. The stress of the tension and possible passive aggressiveness between your kids and your man may be the starting point of a dwindling relationship, even if you feel you and him are strong enough to handle it. Let's say you and your man have a very strong relationship and feel you can battle anything that comes ahead. Then you two, as the adults, should find ways to resolve this tension between the kids and him now and not wait until after the move. Now, if there is no tension and you are simply observing that communication seems to be lacking between your kids and your boyfriend, then you, as the better communicator should explain to him that if you are going to take this step, he will need to try a bit harder to get to know your kids. Remember, he is not just moving in, he is sharing a life with you, which means everything that comes with it.

Q. I am an independent single mom who has her own three-story house, a great career, and a great group of friends. I am pretty content, but most people think I am in denial since I am not in a relationship. Do you think this is true?

A. Since you and I have never met, it is difficult to determine if you are, considering I do not know how you act, what you normally would say, or the feelings you express when you are in denial. Nonetheless, the best way to determine if you are is if after you have taken inventory of your life and you still feel good, then you are not in denial. You are just happy with your life without a partner to share it with. Balance is definitely the key to true satisfaction, so love and connection to another is an essential process to undergo, but being without a partner doesn't mean you are not addressing the "love" part in your life. If you have left time on a routine basis to serve compassionately, to spend with a companion, to meditate on your connection with others, to treat yourself and others with love, to open your heart to whatever comes, you are addressing your love life indeed! So you are living the balanced life. If after everything you have accomplished things still do not feel right to you, even if you have everything you have hoped for and dreamed on becoming and doing, then it could be that you do desire to share all of it with someone. This doesn't mean you are unhappy, but balance is important. If you are in a great relationship, feel insecure, and that you are really missing something, it is not him. It is what you could be doing passionately, while he is gone. On the other hand if, you have a great career, money and all the luxuries in life and then you go on vacation and you still feel like you're missing something, it is not your job. It may be the connection you yearn for. You see, when you seek too much of something, you may be neglecting another. If you try just to work on all areas, then you may be successful in every one of them beyond your wildest dreams.

Q. I am currently pregnant and I am about to do this alone. Am I going to need to go on welfare?

A. It is ironic how many of the questions I receive are in reference to whether or not someone who has a child will need to go on welfare. Without knowing all aspects of your financial life and without being aware of who is and who is not supporting you, I cannot tell you. If you do have some support try to talk to someone to give you an objective opinion. That person can probably give some insight about how you are currently handling your current cash flow or paychecks that will enable you to decide if that type of assistance is right for you. I know that since it is available, the easiest decision would be to go for it. Remember, however, that you eventually want to get to a place where you are not dependent on this type of assistance in order for you to get into the habit of being self sufficient in case the criteria to be qualified changes. There are resources you can tap into. You just have to make the effort to find them.

Q. Can I choose a religion for my child?

A. My thought on that is that you have to decide for your child until she is able to truly decide on her own. However, if you and your family's religion dictate otherwise, you will need to decide if religion is crucial in your decisions while raising your child. Tell your child, when he or she is old enough, about your authentic experiences with this religion.

Q. Dating doesn't seem to be easy for me. Once a guy discovers I have a child, he either doesn't call back or his behavior seems to change a little. Does being a single mom in the dating scene have to be this hard?

A. It doesn't, however, you may meet some men who, no matter what, do not want children or want to be involved with someone who has children whom he does not father. This is why it is a good idea to just tell them straight from the start or at least do not wait too long. The advantage is you will know from the get go if a man has these rules for himself. A lot of people, men and women, wait to tell their dating partners believing that with time it won't matter since the relationship would have grown strong. A lot of people are then surprised to find out the news and the lie becomes a deal breaker. You might as well weed out the ones not the least bit interested in having kids or raising your children. There are some men who will stick around regardless, since they feel you may be worth it, they fall in love with the kids, or they see you and the kids becoming the family he has never had. Just work on renewing yourself and you will attract the right partner someday, probably because you have got your home life together. Then he will not be so worried that he will have to play rescue nanny or super father figure, when he may not have any idea what being a father is like himself.

Q. I am dating a single dad, but I have kids myself. I would like to know at what pace should I proceed? Oh, I forgot to tell you that the mother ran out on him and the two kids.

A. Wow! It is difficult for me to imagine how a mother can run out on her kids like that, but I don't know their situation. Whether it happened a long time ago or if it happened last week, it is very hard for children to simply get over their mother leaving. Believe it or not, even if the mother left before when they were babies, before they got a chance to know her, it is probably a daily challenge to see other mothers and their children now that they are older and trying to comprehend why their mommy didn't want them. Either way, you have probably got to be confident in the longevity of your relationship, before becoming a consistent figure in the children's lives. They do not need to get used to "mother figures" walking out over and over again. They may blame themselves, become resentful, or take it out on dad. However they deal with it, it will not be easy for you. The kids may shower you with love and become really excited about you being at their place everyday, but have this discussion with their dad and determine if this is just a fling or if you guys see yourself going somewhere. The future isn't certain, but if you both have the same goal in mind, it is a good starting point for moving forward and establishing some consistency.

Q. My finances are a mess! I can't seem to budget myself and I am living paycheck to paycheck. I am thinking about dating a guy who is willing to take care of my son and me financially. He seems to be doing very well. I wouldn't even need to work full time! I am not really interested in him romantically, though. I am not sure how to move forward with him.

A. Being taken care of financially is a dream come true to many women in most cultures, especially if she doesn't have to work full time or even at all, but I also know women who have made that choice prematurely and currently find themselves "stuck" only playing a wife and mother role, doing very little with their time. I have also seen it the other way around, when women fall for men who have no goals whatsoever and, therefore now "stuck" at a dead end job or still living with their husbands at his parents, when she really wants out. Anything can happen, but I can only tell you that the women I find who seem to be the happiest are the ones who have partners or husbands with goals who have proven their ability to be successful at something. We all need time to "find ourselves," but at a certain age you start to realize that you just want to make money doing what you love. If this financially secure man is not someone you love, you have to weigh what is more important to you: love or security. Why can't you have both? Using him to rescue you from your financial decline is not a good idea. What happens when he has finished paying all your bills? What next? What is your foundation for a good marriage or partnership? Is this fair to him or does he even care? Will he care one day and claim that he has given you more then enough of his years for you to learn to love him and you still can't respond the way he wants? Many great relationships come from being friends first. If you aren't friends and he is simply doing this to win your love, you both may be surprised that the tangible fixes only go so far. Get yourself together financially so you are not in a position to make this choice at any point in your life.

Q. I am thirty-eight years old and a single mom. Since my time is limited, what is the best way I can discover a new talent? I am so tired of doing what I do now.

A. If you find absolutely no satisfaction with what you do now, take the necessary steps to find what you are passionate about, while you still have a job. You have this advantage, unless you are terminated or laid off. At that point you really don't have a choice, but to get on your horse and go. If the issue is that you are just not tapping into what you are passionate about because you don't even know what it is then here is one way to find out. Since creativity comes from inspiration, and inspiration comes from a divine source, you tap into it by allowing yourself routine time to meditate. Studies have shown that people who meditate routinely run into the events and things that happen to support what they love and desire to create. Another way is to step out of your comfort zone. If you play it too safe then, you risk losing opportunities because you are simply too afraid. Nothing positive can come out of fear. If you get out there and initiate, you have made your intention known and the universe will offer you what you are looking for. If you constantly fear change, you will consistently meet with what makes you afraid all the time. That is just the way it is. Many new experiences are scary at first and then you get over it. It is like learning to swim or riding a bike. You will never do it if you don't jump in or get on

Q. I feel like God has blessed me with a supportive family and my child's father has been really responsible and great with her. I don't seem to have a lot of the challenges many others may have. Now I feel like I need to give back. What are some ways I can do that with my limited time?

A. A great way to start is to get your child involved in a community project serving either animals or a population. It will be a way for you and your child to serve together and she could feel like she made a difference, which in turn feels like you did too, since you are her role model. Between all the online charities, shelters, school fundraisers, and "Go Green" projects, I am sure you can find something. Your child's PTA may offer opportunities to get involved, or you can join the board of some nonprofit organization. Also, daily minor acts of kindness can become your community service regimen. I recall one day last week I signaled an elderly lady to turn her car the other direction or she will get a parking ticket. She turned around to see the police officer coming and she was grateful for the tip. You don't have to yell at every cashier for giving you the wrong change and you don't have to always step over broken glass just laying somewhere in the hallway of some building without informing someone who works there or picking it up with tissue yourself. You can even swap your current cell phone for a "green" phone to do your part in getting educated about saving the planet. My own daughter reminded me to stop talking about moving the cement block everyone was aware of covering part of the sidewalk and just to do it.

Q. I would like to stay healthy to preserve my sanity, but it is challenging while shopping for my two kids, since I can't only buy the healthiest stuff for them.   A healthy lifestyle seems to be expensive for both my kids and me.

A. I understand this because, to me, it doesn't make sense that the most affordable items are the ones that contain the highest fat, the most sugar and the worst carbs. Since we can't change the prices ourselves, you have to do your best to balance your meals between the healthy and the well...replacements. Not all pre-packaged or TV dinner meals are bad for you. You just have to read the labels for high sodium, sugar etc... I get the impression that all your healthy meals you buy are for yourself. If I am right then, unless you can afford healthy meals for all, you should probably get your kids in the habit of eating healthy like you now by introducing some of what you eat into their meals. They don't have to eat an all raw veggie and tofu diet like you. You can simply replace their usual pudding cup with a bowl of their favorite fruits. It is good for your meals to stay colorful on your plate. So if your kids don't like asparagus, give them broccoli with some seasoning, or green peas instead. Change it up a bit. Having pizza night once in a while will not kill them, but having pizza every night may hurt their health and your wallet, especially if you are spending the rest of your food money on healthy meals just for yourself.

Q. My sex drive seems to be pretty low. It happened once I became a mom and I feel like I have forgotten how to be sexy. How can I get this back?

A. Do you even *feel* sexy? You can't be sexy if you don't feel it. It is not about forgetting. It's about identifying how sexy you are and naturally expressing it. The extra effort in your wardrobe and appearance doesn't hurt either, although I know women who dazzle it up on a daily basis and cannot seem to achieve the sexy look they are going for because they are so busy being afraid that they are not so they overdo it. If you think you aren't sexy then you are not and that is just the bottom line. When you have confidence, you are your own best friend and who better then your best friend to always make you feel comfortable with who you are? Trying too hard may be hurting you. What also may be decreasing your sex drive is lack of exercise and, thereby lack of energy and flexibility in the bedroom. Also, if you are with a partner who tends to block his communication, or put you down constantly, your sex drive will diminish. Since we women tend to enjoy sex more after we have released our built up emotions by communicating (in a healthy way), the inability to vent or be validated will affect what goes on in the bedroom.

Q. What do you think about starting a single mothers group online?

A. I think it's great, but I don't know if you are aware that there are a plethora of single mother groups online and you may want to have a premise that keeps your group unique, like single mom book clubs etc...I am sure even that one exists. You also want to make sure that the group is not formed as a vendetta against men, married women, or single women without kids. Otherwise, go for it!

References

Shelton, Dr. Herbert. *Human Life: Its Philosophy of the Principles and practices of Orthopathy*, Oklahoma City, Oklahoma: How To Live Pub CO. 1979

U.S. Census Bureau *Custodial Mothers and Fathers and Their Child Support, Consumer Income* August 2007

U.S. Department of Labor Bureau Labor of Statistics. *Consumer Expenditure Survey* 2007 April 2009 www.bls.gov

NOTES

Sunny Fungcap

www.ingramcontent.com/pod-product-compliance
Lightning Source LLC
Chambersburg PA
CBHW021158010426
R18062100001B/R180621PG41931CBX00027B/47